barefoot and in the Kitchen

barefoot and in the Kitchen

vegan recipes for you

ASHLEY ROWE

Barefoot and in the Kitchen
Vegan Recipes for You

by Ashley Rowe

Illustrated by Ashley Rowe
Edited by Adam Gnade
Designed by Joe Biel

Recipes belong to their respective authors

Published by:

Microcosm Publishing
112C S. Main St.
Lansing, KS 66043-1501
&
636 SE 11th Ave.
Portland, OR 97214

www.microcosmpublishing.com

ISBN 978-1-934620-55-7
This is Microcosm #76111

First Published July 1, 2012
First printing of 5,000 copies

Distributed by Independent Publisher's Group, Chicago

Contents

Introduction:
Cook Your Own F***in' Life!

I started cooking as a teenager, when I became vegetarian—and soon vegan, after doing research into factory farming and animal rights. I'll spare you the gory details of what animals go through to be turned into food, since it's easy to read up on elsewhere, and anyway, if you're interested in vegan cooking you probably know a bit about this unsavory topic already. Instead, I want to focus on all the awesomeness that my decision to go vegan has brought to my life over the last decade or so.

I learned to prepare foods that I liked without all the animal products I was used to—no small challenge, given that I've always been a picky eater, and at that time there were only a fraction of the vegan specialty products we have today. It was a challenge, but as I went along, flipping through cookbooks and websites trying to get inspired, I realized something: It was also fun. A lot more fun than I'd been expecting! And less difficult than I'd feared, too. In fact, vegan cooking was effing rad!

I come from a background of DIY/punk ethics, which told me that not only was it my responsibility to take care of my needs and wants I should also do so as ethically as possible. More importantly, it told me that I could do this however I saw fit and didn't have to follow what other people said was the "right" way to cook or enjoy food. I could throw stuff together, make things up, and mash up different recipes however I wanted—totally inspiring, and a great way to get into something you have

no clue how to do! It wasn't long before I fell in love with food and cooking, and joyfully started doing it my way.

Through my cooking, I've been able to eat cheaper and more healthfully, and have more control over what I put into my body. It wasn't always about health for me—and that's still only a small part of it—but being vegan has definitely helped me to feed myself stuff that is better for my body than anything I ate before. I've always been a picky eater but going vegan opened up my eyes to so many new vegetables and other plant foods that I didn't know about or thought I didn't like, like kale and quinoa. It's certainly possible to subsist as a "junk food vegan" on incidently vegan crap like Oreos and vegetarian Hormel chili—and it's nice to have those things around on occasion—but it's more interesting and satisfying to experience the possibilities in making your own food. Also, did I mention cheaper? Buying unprocessed food can be a small miracle for your grocery bill.

My cooking connected me with people in ways I never expected. About five years into my veganism, I put together a zine of my favorite recipes. That zine was *Barefoot and in the Kitchen #1*. I initially made thirty copies. Little did I know that after taking it to shows and bookfairs and zine symposiums and advertising it on the internet how many visits to the copy shop I was bound for. I went through hundreds of copies and made three more issues! I've gotten to trade for other people's zines, talk to kids who were new to veganism, share recipes with tons of friends and family, hook up with some great zine distributors—including Microcosm—and all in all have an amazing experience. And I've been lucky enough to have that experience culminate now in this book you hold in your hands.

So what's up with this book, anyway? It's mostly recipes, sure—it's a cookbook, after all. But I hope it's something more, too. Following old-school zine traditions, I've filled it with art and comics and little asides. I'm proud to be able to share a handful of guest recipes by some talented friends scattered throughout the book!

I hope you enjoy what you find here, and are able to change it, expand it, and make it your own. In the spirit of DIY ethos, it's time for you to get out there and cook your own fuckin' life!

It's my hope that you will have found your way to this book as new-to-cooking, new-to-veganism, or both. If you fall into any of these categories, welcome! You're in the right place, and I'm happy to have you.

I have no formal culinary background myself, so everything I know about food and cooking is from years spent reading cookbooks, scouring the internet for info on ingredients and techniques and, mostly, a lot of trial and error. Mostly trial, but some error too. I'm telling you this because I think coming to the world of vegan cooking with no background—with fresh eyes and an open mind—is rad, and I want you to be excited about what you've got in your future, rather than intimidated by it.

To help generate excitement and quash intimidation, I've put together some short primers on some of the ingredients and techniques used in this book, as well as a little peak into my personal philosophy of cooking. Some of this stuff is probably relevant to the "initiated" too, so I encourage you to read on!

A Few Things About Cooking:

• You're going to mess things up occasionally. It's cool. Lots of times your food will be salvageable. Sometimes, it's okay to start again.

• Try to chop each ingredient into evenly-sized chunks. If you're making home fries and you have some giant pieces of potato and some little tiny ones, you're going to end up with some crunchy, undercooked bites and some mushy, overdone ones (and maybe a few cooked juuuust right)! The pieces don't have to be perfect, just approximate. Don't stress! Just be aware as you chop.

• Don't burn stuff! Keep an eye on it, turn down heat if you need to, and stir it so that no one part gets direct heat for too long. Seems obvious, but watch your food while it cooks. This can be hard if you've got a bunch of things going on at once, but chances are you'll get more comfortable with kitchen multitasking the more you do it, and you can recruit a friend to help out. That's more fun anyway.

• Spice to taste. That's right! Most of these recipes, and about all other recipes you'll come across, give you measurements for the amount of seasoning to add to your dish. These are guidelines, and they're often excellent, but don't be afraid not to follow them exactly. The food you're preparing should be as delicious as possible to you, so go wild.

• Similarly, don't hesitate to add or subtract whole parts of recipes, or mish-mash different ones together! I suggest trying the recipe as-is at least once to get a feel for it, but like I said, this food is for you and can be made exactly how you'll enjoy it most.

• Read the recipe all the way through before cooking. Remember being told this about assignments in school? My chemistry teacher used to drill this into us. Like a chemistry experiment, your cooking experiment will go smoother if you know what to expect and what you're trying to do before you begin. Also, this book is full of "ridiculously useful tips" to help you along as you go through the recipes, as well as references to the various guides and glossaries, which you may want to read before you start cooking.

• Think about presentation. This is by no means the most important, but once you're comfortable with your cooking, it's nice to make it look nice. "Plating," as you will call it once you've graduated to fancy-pants pseudo-chef status, is one of the main things separating reasonably-priced restaurant meals from crazy-expensive restaurant meals. Might as well go for the gold and make your DIY home-cooked meal look like it came from a restaurant you could never afford to eat at, right? Sounds fun to me!

• Be aware of food allergies. If you're cooking for other people, there's a possibility that one or more guests will have an allergy or sensitivity and need to avoid certain foods. It's important to know this stuff, so polling your friends and family to make sure you have a good grip on their dietary needs and restrictions is the way to go. Fortunately, vegan food bypasses several major allergens—dairy, eggs, fish and shellfish—but there are common ones you'll have to be on the lookout for. Some people have an allergy to wheat gluten. Many others have a milder intolerance, which precludes them from eating the obvious bread and seitan, but also the less obvious items from barley to processed oats and some brands of soy sauce. Other common allergies include soy, peanuts, and tree nuts. Some folks are allgergic to sunflower seed oil or strawberry seeds! Be careful to look at the packaging of processed foods. A lot of things will say "made in a facility that also processes milk ingredients." Depending on the severity of their allergy, some people will have to avoid foods that may have come into contact with allergens. Even small amounts of allergens or intolerances can ruin someone's day so be cautious and communicative. You can never be sure you're gonna feed your guests right unless you have a check-in, so talk to them about it! They'll love you and your delicious cooking all the more for it.

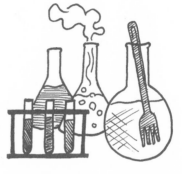

COOKING = SCIENCE!

Ingredients Primer

• *Egg replacer:* There are many substitutes for eggs in baking and cooking, ranging from applesauce and oil to dry powders that you mix with water. Each type has its applications (and you can easily research all the different options online), but the two I tend to use most often are mashed ripe bananas and Ener-G brand powdered egg-replacer. Bananas work well in some baked goods and pancakes, where their flavor will compliment whatever you are making rather than clash with or overwhelm it. When using bananas, it's best to have a very ripe one which can be mashed thoroughly either in your hands or with a fork. One medium sized banana will substitute for two eggs in a recipe. Ener-G is a brand name product that can be bought at natural foods stores or online. It works well in a variety of contexts—all you have to do is mix it with the prescribed amount of water (the box will tell you!) and beat the hell out of it 'til it's foamy. Then add it right into your recipe!

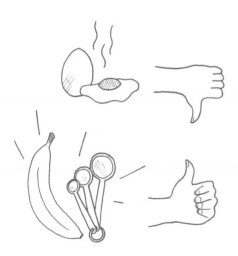

• *Margarine:* There are different types of margarine available, but watch out, because the majority of them contain dairy! It's a real bummer, but there's good news: You've got a number of vegan options, ranging from organic and non-hydrogenated, to conventional, mainstream supermarket fare. My favorite is Earth Balance, which comes in both tub and stick form (great for baking!) and several different varieties including organic and soy-free, if that's how you do things. It's also non-hydrogenated, which is your healthiest bet and gives it a leg-up over most other margarines. Other popular brands that are vegan as of this writing and will do if they are all you can get your hands on are Nucoa, Blue Bonnet Light, and Smart Balance Light. Don't be fooled, because regular old Smart Balance and Blue Bonnet margarines are not vegan. Always be careful and check the ingredients!

• *Nutritional yeast:* You know you're a vegan when the idea of sprinkling yeast over three fourths of the food you eat not only sounds not-insane, but is reality. You may never get to this stage with nutritional yeast—though, never say never!—but even if you don't, it definitely has its uses. It's got an excellent savory, slightly cheesy, slightly nutty flavor, which lends itself to cheese sauces and other recipes. It's high in B12, which is hard to find in vegan sources of and is important to your diet! People call it nooch (n₅ch?), or nut yeast, which I think makes it sound super-unappealing, but don't beat yourself up if you ask someone to pass the nut yeast for your popcorn. It's cool. You're in good company.

• *Tofu*: If you've been vegan or vegetarian for any amount of time, chances are you are well-acquainted with tofu in at least some of its various forms. If not, have no fear! It's true, tofu can be sort of unappealing—or downright gross—when prepared badly, but there's good news: Tofu takes on any flavor you give it and once you know the different types and their applications, you're bound for success!

• *Silken/soft tofu*: Silken tofu is its own type of tofu—the softest and most gelatinous form. It often comes in an aseptic pack, which means that it's in kind of a box rather than packed in water in plastic. This is what you want to use for blending into soups, or for something like a mousse or tofu pie. This is not what you want to use for something you want pieces of tofu in, like a scramble or fried tofu.

• *Medium firm tofu*: Some people like this, and in your cooking you may well find any number of applications for it, but I rarely use it myself. This is useful for something like the tofu ricotta in the Stuffed Shells recipe, which benefits from the tofu being somewhat soft and smooth, but not totally, like silken tofu would be. In general, I say "go big or go home." Er, I mean, "go soft or go extra firm."

• *Extra or super firm*: The best tofu! Or at least the best at what it does. Drain it well and fry it in cubes or slabs or strips, or crumble it for a tasty tofu scramble. I like my tofu as firm as possible. You can shop around to find a brand that's your desired firmness, since they're each a little bit different. Here in California I like the Wildwood brand.

Speaking of draining tofu, let's talk about that for a second. For pretty much everything but the aseptic packed soft tofu, you're gonna want to get as much water out of it as possible. You have a few options for doing this, which range from pressing—setting under a plate with something heavy on top for fifteen-thirty minutes—to wrapping it in cheesecloth or paper towels and squeezing with your hands for a minute or so. Be gentle with the squeezing, unless you're going to be crumbling the tofu anyway!

• *Seitan/Vital wheat gluten*: Vital wheat gluten is a flour derived from the protein portion of wheat, which can be prepared as seitan, an excellent meat substitute. To make seitan, wheat gluten is combined with water, kneaded, then boiled in a flavored broth. Once prepared, seitan can be baked, stir-fried, or pretty much anything else you'd do with a savory protein. You can buy pre-made seitan by itself or in the form of many different types of fake meats at natural foods stores and vegetarian restaurants, but it's much more fun and economical to make your own. Vital wheat gluten can be purchased in the bulk section, or sometimes in boxes, at most natural foods stores, or online.

• *Soymilk* and other milk substitutes: I always say soymilk in my recipes, but this can mean rice or almond milk pretty much interchangeably if you're trying to avoid soy, or don't have any soymilk. All the non-dairy milks have slightly different flavors and properties, so if you're not familiar with them, try out a few and see which is your preferred one, then go with it!

• *Sticky rice*: Sticky rice (or "glutinous rice", a reference to its sticky qualities) is basically what it sounds like: a type of short-grained sweet white rice that is sticky when cooked. The type I have says Thai Sticky Rice on the bag, but you can look for anything that says sticky rice or glutinous rice for use in the Mango Sticky Rice recipe in this book.

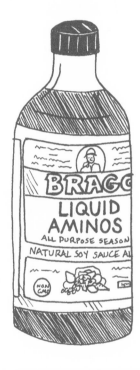

• *Bragg Liquid Aminos*: Commonly referred to as "Bragg's," this is a name brand product made from soy beans containing a whole bunch of essential and non-essential amino acids. It is salty but milder than soy sauce, and can be used in most of the same ways as soy sauce. I like its mellower taste and put it on lots of different foods to give them a salty-savory depth.

• *Vegetable broth*: Can be made fresh, bought packaged, or made using dried bouillon cubes. I usually use bouillon based on convenience, and the fact that it takes up a small amount of space in your cabinet and stores for a long time.

• *Brussels Sprouts*: Totally eat Brussels sprouts! Don't be fooled by their bad reputation—they are delicious! I nominate them vegetable of the year. Sometimes people fuck them up by over-cooking them, especially by boiling, which makes them stinky and not very delicious. But it's so easy to prepare them well, and when they're prepared well... oh man. Also, have you ever seen how they grow? It's amazing! If you have internet access, look up pictures right now.

• *Pine Nuts*: Fun fact! On occasion, a small minority of pine nuts may cause the eater to experience what is known as "pine mouth." A couple days after eating the pine nuts, the eater experiences a strong, bitter metallic taste that is unpleasant and can last up to two weeks. Don't be scared though—lord knows I eat a lot of pine nuts, and I've never experienced any of this craziness. If you do get it, it doesn't cause any lasting harm and will go away on its own. And you'll now know what it is and won't worry that you have a brain tumor or something.

I feel like I'm not doing a great job of selling you on pine nuts, but they are extremely delicious and have a unique and wonderful texture. They are expensive, but wonderful if you can acquire them. They can sometimes be substituted with something else, like walnuts, as in this book's pesto recipe.

- *Quinoa:* It's pronounced "keen-wah." It looks crazy and is confusing if you've never heard it spoken. If you have never had quinoa, you are in for a treat! It's an amazing little seed, which looks and acts like a grain, though it is not. It cooks and can be used like rice, and is a rare complete protein that also boasts fiber and iron.

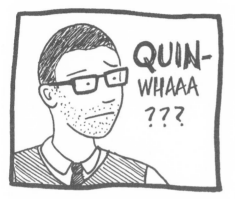

- *Textured vegetable protein (TVP):* A dried protein derived from soy and other plant sources. You can buy it in bulk or packaged at natural foods stores. It can be reconstituted with very hot water or broth to turn it into a chewy, ground beef texture. It has little flavor on its own, and will take on any flavor you give it. I like to use TVP in chili and meaty pasta sauces.

- *Chocolate:* Tons of chocolate and chocolate products contain dairy and thus aren't vegan. But this doesn't have to be the case! Chocolate itself comes from the seeds of the cacao tree and is vegan until someone adds milk or whey to it. It is possible to find vegan chocolate chips, chocolate bars, and cocoa powder—all you have to do is look! A lot of semi-sweet chocolate chips are dairy-free, and you can often find a vegan dark chocolate bar if you read the ingredients. Almost all unsweetened cocoa powder is vegan, but again check the ingredients to be positive.

Besides dairy, there are ethical issues with chocolate. The cocoa industry can be brutal—including forced and child labor in many parts of the world. Buying fair trade chocolate whenever possible can prevent you from supporting these practices, and doing research on which companies to avoid will also help. As always, it's important to know what you're putting in your body and who and where it is coming from!

- *Pasta:* It's kind of a common misconception that a lot of pasta isn't vegan. Most dried pastas you find at the store are vegan—unless they're egg noodles, in which case that's obvious. Soft, fresh-made pastas are where you're likely to get in trouble, as most do contain eggs.

Other than that, you've got your choice of pastas, including whole wheat! I am a whole wheat convert. I used to dislike it, since it is chewier and grainier, but I've gotten used to it and now prefer it. It's a more substantial and much better for you. Regular or whole wheat will work in any of the recipes in this book.

*Bonus tip! Always salt your water, and bring it to a full boil before adding in pasta to cook it!

- *Onion powder:* I don't know what it is about onion powder, but I think it might be magic. No matter what the dish is, if you are making something savory, chances are it will be improved by a dash of onion powder. Try it, that's all I'm saying.

- *Garbanzo beans (Chickpeas):* You can use canned—which I usually do! I'm not above it and you don't have to be either!—or dried, which you have to soak for several hours and then cook.

• *Vanilla*: Please try to use pure vanilla extract and not vanilla "flavoring" or, even worse, "imitation vanilla flavoring." It's slightly more expensive, but it makes a noticeable difference. Trust me, you want your food to taste like fresh vanilla and not a chemical substitute. Read the packaging carefully.

• *Tahini*: Tahini is to sesame seeds what peanut butter is to peanuts. It's used a lot in Mediterranean and Middle Eastern cooking, and is the main ingredient in tahini sauces on falafel sandwiches. It makes great sauces and dressings, and is a natural with lemon juice and garlic. One weird thing is that when you start to stir water into it to thin it down, it'll get thicker and sort of gummy for a minute. Don't be alarmed! Just add a little more water and keep stirring. It'll end up doing exactly what you'd expect.

• *Kale*: Kale is so good for you it's ridiculous. It's a "leafy greenie," as my friend Tucker would say, so you know it's got good potential to be both healthy and delicious. Don't overcook it or it will become too wilty and sad. Also, I like to take the center "vein" out before cooking, because it's pretty tough and crunchy.

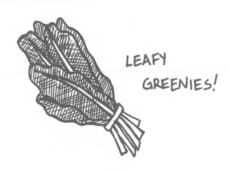

LEAFY GREENIES!

Glossary of Cooking Terms:

-*Beat*: Usually when I call for beating ingredients together in a recipe, I mean for you to use one of my favorite tools—an electric hand mixer!—to combine quickly and thoroughly. In baking, beating also introduces tiny air bubbles, which keep cakes and breads fluffy and cookies chewy and light. Often you can achieve almost the same effect with just your hand and a whisk or large spoon, but it's a lot more work and time to do it that way. But if you get into the habit of beating by hand, you'll build massive forearms!

-*Blend*: I'm positive you know what this means, but I'm including it here to give you some options! For most of our blending purposes, a food processor would probably work best, but not everyone has a food processor (that shit is expensive!). But you can always use your trusty old blender—it may take a little longer and a few more scrape-downs, but it'll get you there in the end. Or, if you're dealing with soup or something and you're a fancy-pants with an immersion blender, go ahead and use that.

-*Dice*: To dice is to chop into medium small (usually a half inch or so) pieces that are roughly cube-ish in shape. Not as intense as mincing, just sort of a nice, everyday kind of chop.

-*Knead*: You probably know about kneading dough for bread and such, but in this book, you'll also use this technique for making seitan and a couple other things. Kneading involves stretching, pressing, and rolling dough on a flat surface to warm and stretch the gluten within it, making the finished product strong and elastic (both good things!).

-*Mince*: Cut it up real small! Garlic is often minced, and I mince ingredients like shallot when it's going in a dressing or sauce and I don't want big crunchy chunks of it. Chop it with a big knife until it's turned into super small pieces.

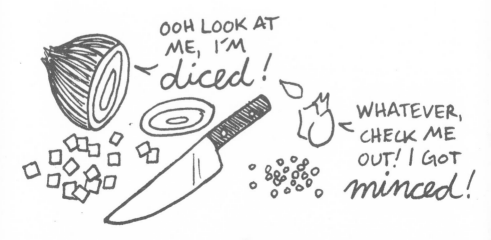

OOH LOOK AT ME, I'M *diced!*

WHATEVER, CHECK ME OUT! I GOT *minced!*

-*Reduce*: To reduce something's liquidity is what it sounds like: reducing the amount of liquid it contains to thicken and concentrate what remains. Heating juice, vinegar, or a sauce over low-medium heat for awhile will reduce it by letting out water as steam. Watch it and stir every so often to prevent burning!

-*Roast*: Roasting is one of my favorite cooking methods. It's easy and does a great job bringing out the deep, delicious flavor in vegetables. Toss whatever you like in a bit of oil, add some seasonings, and stick it in the oven. You can get more complicated if you like, but there's no need. I like to roast at a high temperature (usually 425), to speed cooking and get that nice done-on-the-inside, kinda-crispy-on-the-outside sort of appeal. Sit back and stir every ten to fifteen minutes to avoid burning or sticking!

*Bonus tip! I like to line whatever oven-safe pan I'm using to roast with tinfoil or parchment paper. This makes cleanup easy—you better believe there's nothing I hate more than having to clean a giant casserole pan that's got veggie pieces and burnt balsamic baked on!

-*Sauté*: Sautéing vegetables allows them to be cooked quickly with a small amount of oil. You'll notice a lot of the recipes in the book call for onion and garlic to be sautéed together as the base for a sauce or soup. You'll want a shallow pan, fairly high heat, and to pay attention and stir your veggies around often to make sure they cook evenly and don't burn.

-*Sift*: Sifting is a great way to get clumps out of dry ingredients like flour or powdered sugar. Passing these through the metal screen of a sifter will ensure you don't end up with an unexpected lump of dryness in your baked goods that bursts when you bite into it and bums you the hell out.

-*Simmer*: To simmer a liquid, bring it to a boil and then immediately reduce your heat. Simmering involves cooking a sauce or liquid ingredient over low-medium heat for a relatively long time to bring together flavors (as in a tomato sauce), or sometimes to reduce the liquid content.

-*Whisk*: Use a, uh, whisk to stir briskly and combine. If there's no whisk in sight and you're working with dry ingredients, grab a fork!

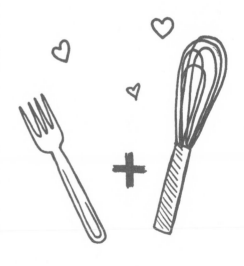

Superior Pasta Salad

The perfect food to take with you—to work, to the beach, to the anarchist bookfair—because it's fine sitting around a little bit, and is good warm or cool. Also, you can put whatever you want in it, though I wouldn't have given you this list of ingredients if I didn't think they were the best! Throw a potluck just so you can serve this.

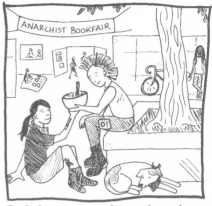

Serves: 4-8

1 16oz. package of pasta*
2 medium carrots, sliced into thin rounds
1/2 medium red onion, finely chopped
1/2 cup fresh chopped basil
1 clove garlic, minced
1/3 cup pine nuts
1/2 cup sliced black olives
3/4 cup kidney beans
2 Tbsp Tbsp olive oil
1 Tbsp balsamic vinegar
2 tsp lemon juice
salt and pepper to taste
generous pinch of nutritional yeast (optional)

Cook the pasta according to the package—you'll probably end up boiling it in salted water for around ten minutes. Once cooked, drain and rinse it with cold water until almost room temperature. Return it to your pot, or a large mixing bowl, and stir in one Tbsp of your olive oil to coat it so it doesn't turn into a sticky noodle mass.

Add in all your chopped veggies, basil, and pine nuts and mix. Toss with the rest of the oil, lemon juice, balsamic, and spices. Keep tasting it and add more of whatever makes it most delicious to you. Serve at room temperature or out of the fridge!

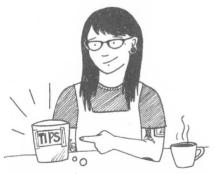

*Ridiculously Useful Tip: Pick any shape pasta you want, with some exceptions that go without saying. But just 'cause, I will tell you anyway: nothing long and thin like spaghetti or fettuccine (duh!). Stick to the little guys like penne or fusili. Or bow ties—cute!

Don't-Fuck-It-Up Guacamole

You'd be shocked how many people and places fuck up guacamole. Cucumber? Why? Sour cream? Barf. It's a handful of fresh ingredients. Respect it for its simple deliciousness and move on.

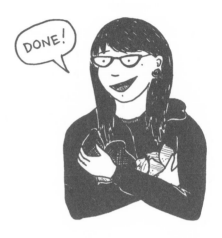

Serves: Who knows? Depends what you use it for and how much you love avocado

2 ripe avocados
1 1/2   Tbsp lime juice (from a couple limes)
1 clove garlic, minced extra small
3   Tbsp minced red onion
salt, to taste

Mince your garlic and onion and add to the avocado innards you've scraped into a bowl. Mash with a fork 'til it starts to get all blended and creamy. Stir in lime juice and add salt to taste.

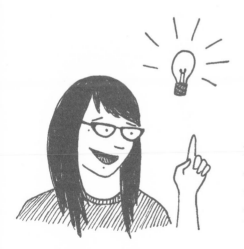

Ridiculously Useful Tip: If you're going to be storing this in the fridge, put plastic wrap directly on it (like, touching the guacamole, not hovering above it uselessly at the top of the bowl). The less air that touches it, the greener it'll stay.

Broccoli Rice Au Gratin

I'm not 100% sure what "au gratin" means, but I'm thinking it's something like "delicious"—I mean unhealthy. But delicious! Fortunately, this recipe delivers all the delicious without all the unhealthy—what a bargain!

Serves: 4
1 1/2 cup uncooked rice (I prefer brown)
3 cup water for cooking the rice
2 crowns of broccoli
1/2 cup soymilk (can be replaced with water in a pinch)
1/3 cup nutritional yeast
1 1/2 Tbsp flour
2 Tbsp olive oil
1 Tbsp Bragg's Liquid Aminos
1/2 tsp garlic powder
1 tsp onion powder
 salt to taste

I bet you know how to cook rice. Maybe you even have a rice cooker. Either way, put the rice and water together (two:one) and cook for twenty minutes or until it's done. Chop the broccoli fairly small (include the stalks if you want—or not!) and steam (using the rice-steam?!) until it is your desired firmness or mushiness.

The rest of this shit is going to make a sauce. Mix it all together, starting with the oil and flour, then add everything else. Pour it over the hot broccoli and rice and mix well. Amazing!

Chocolate Chip Cookies

I know these are "just" chocolate chip cookies, okay? But let me tell you, this one time someone I didn't know came up to me and said she made these all the time and her boyfriend doesn't like sweets but eats them like crazy. So there.

Makes: about 2 dozen

2 1/4 cup flour
1 tsp baking soda
3/4 tsp salt
1 cup (2 sticks) margarine, softened
3/4 cup sugar
3/4 cup brown sugar
2 eggs' worth of egg replacer
1 tsp vanilla
1 tsp baking soda
1 1/2 cup chocolate chips

Preheat your oven to 350.

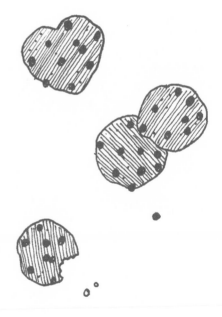

Mix together the margarine, sugars, and vanilla and then cream with an electric mixer. Add in your egg replacer and beat well. Sift (or whisk) together your dry ingredients, and stir into the wet mixture. The dough will be a little squishy (not in a gross way!). If it seems way too wet, add in a couple extra Tbspsps of flour. Mix in the chocolate chips!

Form the dough into golf-ball-sized balls and flatten into discs. Bake on a cookie sheet an inch or so apart for nine to eleven minutes.

Amazing Meaty Lasagna

This recipe looks more labor-intensive than it is, but even if it took five hours and $70 to make, I think it would be worth it. That's how much fun it is to trick meat-eating friends into enjoying a thoroughly meaty, 100% cruelty-free version of a normally very un-vegan dish. Also, it makes great leftovers and you can freeze slices to heat up at a later date!

Serves: 8

1 large box (1 lb) lasagna noodles

For the meaty sauce:
2 12oz. packages vegan ground "beef"
1 medium onion, chopped
4 cup pasta sauce (out of a jar or homemade—both fine!)
4 cloves garlic (or more!), minced
3 Tbsp olive oil
Up to 1 tsp each: dried basil, oregano, thyme
salt and pepper to taste

For the white sauce:
1/2 cup (1 stick) vegan margarine
5 Tbsp flour
2 cup soymilk
salt to taste

Preheat oven to 375 and cook lasagna noodles in a large pot of salted water according to directions on the box. Once cooked, the noodles can sit in some cool water (so they don't stick) until they're needed to assemble the dish.

For the meat sauce, start by sautéing the onion and garlic in the olive oil for five or six minutes until soft in a large pan. Crumble in the veggie meat and add the pasta sauce. Add the herbs and spices and let simmer on low heat for about thirty minutes to let all the flavors mix. Stir often!

Prepare your white sauce when the noodles and meat sauce are ready. To do this, melt the margarine over medium heat and whisk in the flour. Once a paste has been formed, add the soymilk, stirring the whole time. Keep stirring over low-medium heat until the sauce thickens into a good consistency (creamy and thick, but not too thick), about five minutes. FYI: You can add more soymilk to the mixture, but once soymilk has been introduced you can't add flour, so combine slowly!

Lightly grease a large lasagna/casserole pan, and place enough of your cooked noodles on the bottom to cover it (probably four). Pour one third of the white sauce over the noodles and spread to coat evenly. Spread half of the meaty sauce over the noodles and white sauce. Make another layer of noodles and spread another third of the white sauce and the rest of the meaty sauce over this. Arrange one more layer of noodles on the top and spread the remaining white sauce over the top of the lasagna.

Cover the dish with aluminum foil and bake for thirty minutes. Let cool as long as possible before eating (at least ten minutes). This part sucks. It smells good and you'll want to eat it, but you have to wait! It needs time to solidify or when you try to cut and serve it it'll be a big mess.

You'd-Never-Know-It-Was-Vegan Gravy

Who needs turkey fat or gizzards to make gravy? What are gizzards, anyway? Why not celebrate your holiday without taking a life, huh? Makes sense to me. Pour this over stuffing, mashatatoes, etc., etc.

2   Tbsp margarine
2   Tbsp flour
1 cup vegetable broth (see tips in ingredient primer)
1 tsp nutritional yeast
1/4 tsp poultry seasoning
small squirt of soy sauce or Bragg's Liquid Aminos

Melt the margarine over low-medium heat and whisk in the flour to form a paste (or "roux" if you want to be fancy). Add the nutritional yeast and poultry seasoning, then the veggie broth and Bragg's/soy sauce. Stir constantly for several minutes until the gravy thickens to your desired consistency. It will. Keep stirring.

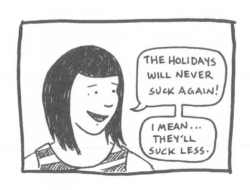

Avocado Milkshake

An avocado milkshake! It's the smartest idea I never thought of! I got this idea from a now-defunct restaurant in San Francisco (R.I.P. Mekong) back in the days when my friend Kathleen was an avocado fan and I was not. She got one, I said "gross!," tried it, and was an instant convert. Seriously, overcome any reservations you may have about this idea. You'll be glad you did.

Serves: 1-2

1 ripe avocado
1 cup soymilk
1 cup ice
2 Tbsp sugar
1 tsp vanilla

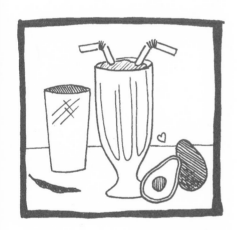

Cut and pit the avocado. Scoop its delicious greenness into a blender with the ice, sweetener, vanilla, and about half the soymilk. Blend the shit out of it, adding soymilk as needed for a creamy, drinkable consistency. Enjoy thoroughly.

Simply the Best
Applesauce

So easy. So good. Shockingly delicious. If you've never had fresh, homemade applesauce before, I guarantee you're going to lose your mind the first time you try this. And it's good hot or cold!

Makes: 4 cups

4 lb apples (around ten medium)*
1/4 cup sugar
1 cup water
1/4 tsp cinnamon
pinch of salt

*I recommend a mix of three fourths Golden Delicious and one fouth Granny Smith apples. Others will work, but trust me, this is ideal.

Peel, core, and roughly chop the apples into one and a half inch pieces.

Put everything except cinnamon in a large pot. Cook covered over medium-high heat for fifteen to twenty minutes until the apples start to break down, stirring occasionally.

When the apples are soft and have begun to mushify, turn off heat, add the cinnamon, and mash with a potato masher or fork. Make it as chunky or smooth as you like!

Spinach Yam Curry

Modeled after one of my favorite dishes from one of my favorite restaurants—I crave their version, but mine makes a good and easy substitute. Best served over rice alongside something salty-savory—teriyaki tofu, perhaps?

Serves: 4

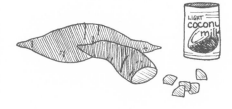

1 (14oz.) can coconut milk (I use light)
2 large yams, yielding ~4 cup 1" cubes
2 cloves garlic, crushed
1 1/2 tsp yellow curry powder*
1/2 tsp onion powder
1 1/2 cup raw baby spinach
salt to taste

*There are lots of curry powder options around, and you're free to find the one that best suits your taste and adjust the amount if you need to. The one I like to use contains: turmeric, cumin, ginger, coriander, fenugreek, garlic, celery seed, cloves, cayenne pepper, caraway seed, white pepper, and mace.

Peel the yams and cut into smallish chunks, about one inch cubed. Simmer everything but the spinach in a covered pan over medium heat for twenty-thirty minutes until the yams are soft and easily cut with a fork. Remove from heat and stir in the spinach. This will make it wilty, but not overcooked. Nice!

Apple Cinnamon Beer Bread

Beer! Turned into a lovely sweet bread in no time! It's the ideal situation. This recipe takes only about 5 minutes of prep time, but an hour of baking, so sit back and enjoy the rest of your six-pack? Or, if that's not how you roll, not to worry! This bread doesn't come out tasting all boozy, and the alcohol burns off in the oven!

Makes: 1 loaf

3 cup all-purpose flour
1/2 cup sugar
1   Tbsp baking powder
1 tsp salt
1 tsp cinnamon
1 small apple, chopped into chunks
1 12oz. bottle of beer*
1   Tbsp melted margarine

*I like to use a hefeweizen, since it's flavorful but also light and somewhat fruity. Anything that's not super-dark or very strong tasting should work though. If you don't have a hefe, try a lager? If you don't give a shit, just pick up something cheap and you should be good to go.

Preheat oven to 375 and grease a loaf pan well.

In a large bowl, whisk together all the dry ingredients. Take one swig of the beer if you want—reducing the liquid by a couple tablespoons is good for this recipe. Pour in the beer and mix with a whisk until it's too sticky. Now it's time to get your hands dirty! Squish and knead with your hands for a few seconds until it's a fairly even consistency, then fold in your apple chunks. The dough will be fairly wet—fear not!

Plop the whole thing into your greased pan and bake for fifty five-sixty minutes. About 50 minutes in, brush or pour the margarine over the top. Your loaf is done when a toothpick comes out clean!

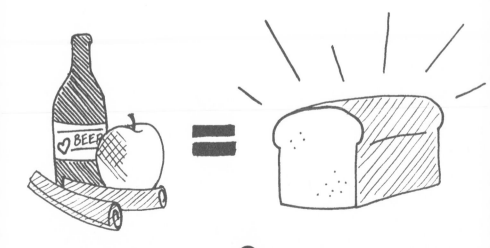

Brussels Sprouts (in a good way!)

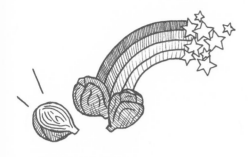

Brussels sprouts are on the receiving end of a lot of shit-talking and, let's face it, it's not fair. They get a bad rap from being overcooked, boiled to the point of no-flavor-all-cabbagey-stink, but when prepared right, they are about the most perfect little packages of deliciousness you can imagine. The perfect side dish for any meal, especially when you need some wintry roasted comfort food!

Serves: 4

1 lb-ish fresh Brussels sprouts
2 Tbsp olive oil
1 Tbsp balsamic vinegar
1/3 cup pine nuts
1/2 tsp salt
pepper (as much as you like)

Preheat your oven to 400.

Cut the tough end off the bottom of the Brussels sprouts and cut each one in half lengthwise. Some outside leaves may fall off. No problem!

In a large casserole pan, coat them in the olive oil, vinegar, salt, and pepper. Don't add the pine nuts yet!

Roast uncovered for thirty- 40 minutes, depending how well-done you want them. Stir every ten minutes or so (maybe a little more frequently toward the end), and add the pine nuts for just the last ten minutes.

Split Pea Soup with Barley

Barley makes a surprisingly awesome addition to this simple, flavorful, filling, great, healthy soup.

Serves: 6-8

2 carrots
1 medium onion
2 stalks celery, with the leafy tops
3 cloves garlic
1 1/2 cup dry split peas
1 cup barley
8 cup water
2   Tbsp soy sauce
salt and pepper to taste

Dice the carrots, celery, and onion, and mince the garlic. Put it all into a large pot with the water, split peas, and soy sauce. Bring the water to a boil and turn the heat down to medium. Cook in your covered pot, stirring occasionally, for fourty five minutes.

Add the barley and take off the lid. Cook uncovered for another thirty minutes. The soup is done when the barley is cooked through and the rest of it is a thick, pleasant mash. Add salt and pepper to taste!

Corn Chowda

Smart Alec's in Berkeley makes the best corn chowder. It's my favorite soup. After many months of trekking out there and coughing up the cash, I decided it was time to make my own. This isn't quite Smart Alec's, but it's pretty damn good and if I can fool myself, so can you. Fool your own self, I mean. And maybe me too.

Serves: 8

5 medium-large potatoes
2 stalks of celery, chopped thin
2 carrots, diced
1 small onion, diced
vegetable broth, several cups
3 cloves garlic
2 cup frozen corn
1/2 cup soymilk
3 Tbsp olive oil
1 Tbsp dill (dried—use less if fresh!)
spices to taste: salt, pepper, onion and garlic powder, chili powder

In a large pot, sauté the garlic, onion, carrots, and celery together in the olive oil until all are beginning to get soft and the onion is translucent (about ten minutes).

Meanwhile, chop the potatoes into bite-sized pieces (I leave the skin on). Once your veggies are pretty much cooked, add the potatoes to your large pot, along with enough broth to cover them, plus about one fourth inch over the top. Boil about ten-fifteen minutes until the potatoes are done.

Take about one third of the veggies and potato bits, minus the broth, and set aside if you want your soup to be chunky (which you do). Then, blend the rest of the soup in batches in a blender or food processor until it's all liquidy.

Once this is all done, pour your blended mixture back into the pot to finish cooking. Add in your un-blended veggies, as well as the corn, and slowly add soymilk until the soup is as thick or thin as you want it.

Keep cooking the soup over medium heat to cook the corn and make it all cohesive while you add the spices. Keep stirring, tasting, and spicing until it has a good consistency and is flavorful and delicious!

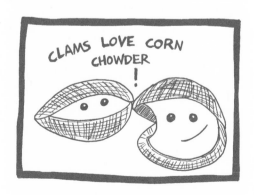

Creamy Asparagus Soup

This soup is ridiculously easy and delicious. It's creamy and rich enough for a winter evening, but not too heavy for, uh, anything other than winter. Serve it in a bread bowl, maybe!

Serves: 8

1 lb asparagus, tough ends chopped or snapped off
1 medium onion, chopped small
5-7 medium red potatoes
a bunch of garlic, like 5 cloves, minced
1/2 package silken tofu
5 cup vegetable broth
1   Tbsp dill (dried—use less if fresh!)
1   Tbsp nutritional yeast, and more to taste
3   Tbsp olive oil
salt and pepper, to taste

Start by sautéing the onion and garlic in olive oil in a large pot over medium heat. Sprinkle in some salt and cook with the lid on for a few minutes until almost salt.

Meanwhile, chop the asparagus into bite-sized pieces. Add to the onion and garlic and cook until it begins to soften.

While this cooks, clean and chop your potatoes into bite-sized pieces. Leave the skin on! Once the asparagus is tender, add the potatoes and vegetable broth to the pot. Stir in the dill and simmer until the potatoes are completely cooked.

When all the veggies are cooked, scoop some out (a cup or two) without the broth, so they won't get blended up and can be added back into the creamy soup later. Set aside.

Add the nutritional yeast and crumble the tofu into the remaining soup. Blend in batches in a blender or food processor until creamy.

Pour back into your pot and add in the veggies you set aside. Warm over medium heat as you add salt, pepper, and more nutritional yeast to taste. Yes!

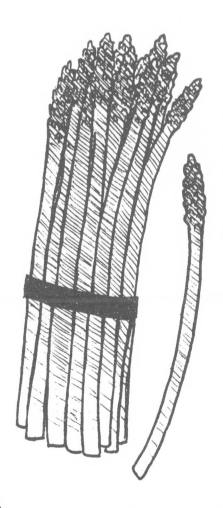

Three Bean Salad with Avocado Vinaigrette

A friend of mine thought to mash some avocado into salad dressing and toss it with a bean salad for a potluck we had. I tried to eat all of it, but other people kept taking their share. I decided to come up with my own dressing recipe, avocado-mash and all, and throw this together myself whenever I want. And not share.

Serves: 4-6

1 (15oz.) can garbanzo beans
1 (15oz.) can kidney beans
1 cup cooked green beans (I use frozen)
1/2 ripe avocado
1/4 medium red onion
2　Tbsp olive oil
2　Tbsp balsamic vinegar
1 clove garlic
salt and pepper to taste

Drain and rinse the garbanzo and kidney beans and combine in a large bowl. Cut or break the green beans into one inch pieces, and defrost if frozen (I do this by running them under warm water for a minute in a colander). Combine with the other beans.

Chop the red onion into small, thin pieces and toss with the beans-and-green-beans. Take one fourth of the avocado (half of your half, get it?), and mix it in with your beans and onion. You can cut it into slices or chunks, or even mash it up. Do whatever you want! It's your salad.

Now make your dressing! Mince the garlic into tiny pieces and stick it into a glass or small bowl. Mash the rest of your avocado and mix it with the oil and vinegar in whatever receptacle you've got your garlic in. Whisk together with a fork until the mixture is creamy and mostly smooth. Add salt and pepper to taste, then toss it with your bean mixture.

Chill in the fridge and serve cold!

Rich Hot Fudge Sauce

This recipe was stumbled upon in my search for the perfect simple fudge (which I also achieved! See page 38). Total necessity, and one that veganism is sorely lacking much of the time. But that is behind us now—make this hot fudge and leave your days of boring, undressed ice cream in the past!

Makes: A bunch! Enough for several sundaes.

1 3/4 cup soymilk
3/4 cup sugar
1/3 cup margarine
1 1/2 cup chocolate chips (1 12oz. bag)
2 tsp vanilla

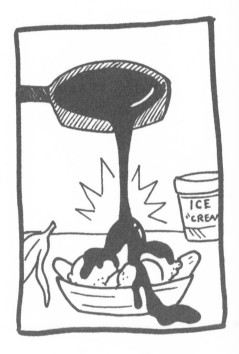

In a medium sized sauce pan over medium heat, bring the soymilk and sugar to a boil. Simmer over low-medium heat for five or six minutes, stirring so it doesn't burn.

In the meantime, combine all your other ingredients in a mixing bowl. Once the soymilk-sugar is through boiling, remove it from heat and stir it into the bowl with the other ingredients. Stir and stir until the chocolate chips and margarine are melted and the mixture has a creamy, even consistency. Serve hot over dairy-free ice cream!

Quinoa Salad with Lemon-Shallot Dressing

This salad has the twin bonuses of being light and also filling. And also the bonus-bonus of being healthy. Read about quinoa in the ingredients primer if the rest of the stuff in this recipe isn't enough to convince you. You can feel free to use this dressing for any of your other salad needs!

Serves: 6

1 1/2 cup dry quinoa, +3 cup water to cook
1 (15oz.) can kidney beans, drained and rinsed
1 carrot chopped thin
a couple big handfuls of baby spinach

Dressing:
1 large garlic clove, minced
one small shallot, about 4   Tbsp minced
3   Tbsp lemon juice (from 1 to 2 lemons)
1   Tbsp olive oil
2   Tbsp tahini
3   Tbsp water
salt to taste

Cook the quinoa with the water over low heat, for about fifteen minutes. Transfer to a large bowl and stick in the fridge or freezer to cool to room temperature. Stir every few minutes until it's cool. You don't want a hot salad, do you? Ew.

Once cool, mix in chopped carrot, spinach, and kidney beans.

Make your dressing in a small glass or bowl by whisking all the ingredients with a fork 'til you've got a creamy, lumpy sauce. It might look crazy for a second, like it's not going to combine, but persevere! Toss it with the salad, making sure to get an even coating! Now you can squeeze some more lemon juice over the salad, or sprinkle it with salt, if you like, and serve!

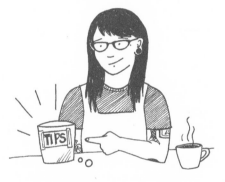

Ridiculously Useful Tip: To cut down on the pain-in-the-ass factor of cooking the quinoa and immediately having to cool it, cook it ahead of time and store it in the fridge!

"Who Cares" Award-Winning Mac and Cheese

This mac and cheese seriously won an award! Second place in a non-vegan mac and cheese bake off. Much to our omnivorous competitors' dismay, our team won the coveted $50 cheese shop gift certificate! Oh, the irony.

This rich mac and cheese is great with steamed broccoli or some BBQ tofu and dark sautéed greens. It's not your everyday weeknight mac. It's more of a dish for a potluck or a dinner party or when you wanna impress the pants off someone. I mean, it's got two sauces, plus bread crumbs!

Serves: 6

16oz. box of pasta, we use Cellentani
dash of paprika (to sprinkle on top)

Cashew Sauce
1 1/3 cup chopped Yukon gold potatoes, about one large potato
1/4 cup chopped carrot, about one medium carrot
1 cup water
1/3 cup raw cashews
1/4 cup raw pine nuts
1/3 cup margarine
1/2 cup nutritional yeast
2 1/2 Tbsp miso
2 Tbsp tahini
2 Tbsp lemon juice (about one juicy lemon)
1 tsp salt
1/2 tsp Dijon mustard

Creamy Sauce
1/2 cup margarine
5 Tbsp flour
2 cups soymilk
1/2 cup nutritional yeast
1/4 tsp turmeric
1/2 tsp salt

Bread Crumb Topping
Use a stale baguette if possible.
You can store any unseasoned breadcrumbs in the freezer in a sealed container. A food processor is best for this, but if you don't have one, a blender will work.

1/2 sweet baguette
2 Tbsp margarine
1/2 cup nutritional yeast
1/4 tsp onion powder

Start a large pot of salted water boiling and preheat oven to 325 F.

Peel and finely chop your potato and carrot. Combine with 1 cup of water in a small saucepan. Cover and cook the potato and carrots on medium-high heat until they're quite soft, about ten-twelve minutes.

Prepare your breadcrumbs by ripping the baguette into one inch chunks. Combine a handful of chunks with the margarine and pulse in your blender or food processor until the crumbs are small and crumbly.

Add the remaining bread chunks. Stir and blend until all the breadcrumbs are small. Add nutritional yeast and onion powder and pulse until combined. Set aside and rinse blender.

In blender combine the cashew and pine nuts. Pulse until the nuts are in small pieces but have not formed a paste. Add the remaining cashew sauce ingredients to the blender, including the softened potato and carrots with the water they were cooked in. Mix with a spoon and then blend away until the sauce is smooth and creamy.

Taste and adjust seasonings to your liking. The sauce should be intensely flavored, since it is going to be combined with the mellow, creamy sauce. Set the cashew sauce aside for now.

Start toasting the breadcrumbs! Toss 'em in a thin layer on a baking sheet covered in parchment or foil and bake for ten-fifteen minutes or until crisp and light gold. You may want to stir them a couple times to ensure even toasting. Set aside to sprinkle over baked mac and cheese.

While breadcrumbs are toasting, start on the creamy sauce.

Melt the margarine in a saucepan on medium heat, and whisk in the flour to make a roux. Once the flour and margarine are thoroughly combined and not lumpy, whisk in the nutritional yeast, salt, and turmeric. Slowly add the soymilk, stirring constantly and scraping the edges and bottom of the pan to combine. Continue to cook over low-medium heat for several minutes, continually stirring, until the sauce thickens to a creamy consistency.

Now combine the two sauces in the blender and blend for fifteen-twenty seconds.

Pour this over your cooked pasta in a baking dish and stir to evenly coat. Cover with foil and bake for twenty five-thirty min.

Sprinkle with breadcrumbs and a dash of paprika and black pepper once everything is out of the oven. Impress the pants off of someone.

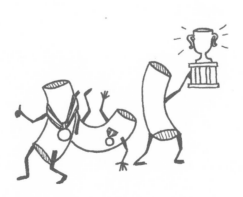

Chocolate Walnut Fudge

So rich and so good. I love to make this fudge and wrap it up in little packets to give as holiday gifts! Everyone loves fudge, and no one has ever been anything less than satisfied with this dairy-free version!

1/2 cup vegan chocolate chips
6 Tbsp margarine (like Earth Balance)
3 cup powdered sugar
1/2 cup cocoa powder
1 tsp vanilla
1/2 cup soymilk
1 cup chopped walnuts (optional, but unless you're allergic you probably want them!)

Grease a 5" x 9" pan with margarine or oil.

In a sauce pan, melt the margarine over low-medium heat and stir in the soymilk. Slowly mix the chocolate chips (a little at a time!), stirring constantly until melted. Stir in all other ingredients except the walnuts, and mix until thoroughly combined and smooth. Remove from heat and quickly mix in the walnuts, then pour into your greased pan. Smooth into an even layer of fudgey deliciousness.

Cover and refrigerate for at least one hour to solidify, but preferably several hours or overnight. Cut into modestly-sized squares (it's rich!) and serve.

Bananana Nut Loaf

This is one of those call-it-a-breakfast-food-and-eat-it-in-the-morning type of situations. Hey, it's got bananas! It's got nuts! That's kind of healthy! This is a veganized version of a much-loved part of my youth. I used to insist on having my own loaf made without the nuts, which I guess you could do too. Or, as long as you're not allergic, you could grow up and enjoy this loaf with all its glorious components intact.

Serves: 2-10 depending how hungry you are and how big a sweet tooth you have

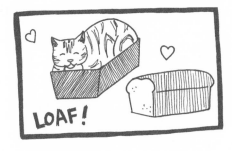

1/2 cup (one stick) margarine
1 1/2 cup sugar
1 1/2 cup bananas* (about 3 medium)
2 cup flour
3/4 cup soymilk
1/2 tsp apple cider vinegar
3/4 tsp baking powder
1/2 tsp baking soda
1/2 tsp salt
1 1/2 tsp vanilla
1 cup chopped walnuts

Preheat your oven to 350.

Start by mixing the vinegar and soymilk together, and setting aside a few minutes for the mixture to get all curdley (you're faking buttermilk here).

Beat together the sugar, margarine, and bananas with an electric mixer. In a separate bowl, whisk together the dry ingredients (not including walnuts!). Add slowly to the wet mixture, stirring to combine.

Add the soymilk mixture and vanilla to the rest and mix well. Last, throw the walnuts in there! Mix 'em in good!

Pour into a large (greased!) loaf pan and bake at 350 for one hour and ten minutes. You can start checking for doneness around fifty five minutes.

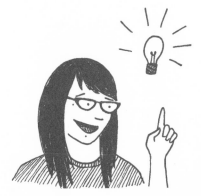

Ridiculously Useful Tip: Use rotten bananas for this recipe—seriously—totally brown bananas, as long as they're not moldy. It sounds gross, but will make your loaf so much better.

Stuffing

I've said it before and I'll say it again: You don't need a dead bird to make a holiday meal. You don't need some kind of tofu or mock-meat product faking a dead bird to make a holiday meal. In my opinion, it's all about the sides; and this one is a classic that's gotten lots of positive feedback over the years. Aren't you glad you don't have to scoop it out of any kind of "cavity" to eat it?

Serves: 6

1/2 cup (one stick) margarine
1 loaf vegan white bread
1 medium onion
4 celery sticks, with leafy tops
1/2 tsp thyme
1/2 tsp onion powder
1 1/2 tsp celery salt
2 1/2 tsp poultry seasoning

Start by melting the margarine in a large pan. Meanwhile, chop the onion and celery small. Add them to the melted margarine and sauté until they are fairly soft. Add about half your spices into the mixture now.

While your veggies are cooking, you can start preparing your bread. Take a couple pieces at a time and dampen them slightly—just slightly!—either with a trickle of water from the tap, or maybe like a spray bottle if you have such a thing. If not, tap water trickle is fine. This is just so the bread doesn't absorb all the margarine the second you crumble it in.

Once all the veggies are cooked and the bread is damp, tear the bread up and throw it into the pan with the veggies. Don't make the pieces quite as small as you imagine the chunks in stuffing to be, as they'll break down into smaller pieces gradually as you stir the mixture.

Stir with a spatula, making sure to break up all the bread and get everything all mixed and evenly coated. Add the rest of your spices, plus more, if you feel so inclined after tasting it. Cook on medium heat 'til it just starts to brown, and serve with vegan gravy!

Perfect Pancakes with Berry Compote

(dedicated to José, the pancake-lover in my life)

Pancake making is an art. Maybe you've heard, "You always have to throw out the first pancake; it never comes out right no matter what you do." Do other people say that or is it just me? Either way, these pancakes are worth the two minutes of practice it takes to get them right. You can feel free to eat them without the compote topping if you like, but why would you want to?

Serves: 5

Pancakes:
1 1/4 cup all purpose flour
3/4 cup whole wheat flour*
1 Tbsp baking powder
1/4 tsp salt
2 cup soymilk
2 Tbsp canola oil
2 Tbsp maple syrup
1 cup frozen or fresh blueberries (optional)

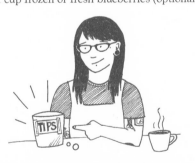

*Ridiculously Useful Tip: You can skip the whole wheat and just use two cups all purpose flour if you don't mind being ever-so-slightly less healthy. I don't recommend using all whole wheat flour, though—the texture gets all crazy!

In a large bowl, whisk together the dry ingredients. Then, pour in wet ingredients and whisk until most lumps are gone (about twenty seconds). Don't overdo it!

Meanwhile, heat up your pan over medium-highish heat. Spoon about three Tbsp of batter onto it at a time, spreading into a nice circle with the back of a spoon. At this point, plop a handful of blueberries around the surface if you want.

The pancake is ready to be flipped with a spatula when bubbles are starting to show on the surface and it looks golden brown when you peak at the underside. Flip and cook the rest of the way, 'til the new underside is golden brown as well. Repeat!

Compote:
2 cup-ish frozen mixed berries
2 tsp sugar
3 Tbsp water
2 tsp lemon juice

*Ridiculously Useful Tip: As you can tell by the ingredient amounts, the compote is not an exact science! Mess around with the amounts 'til you get a flavor and consistency you are happy with.

Combine all ingredients in a small pan over medium heat. Mash the berries with a fork or something as they warm up and thaw. Simmer the compote for several minutes until some of the liquid is reduced out and it's kind of lumpy-syrupy (better than it sounds!). Serve atop your perfect pancakes!

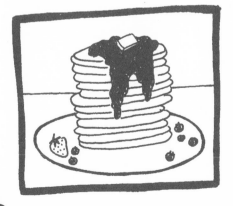

Stuffed Shells

These stuffed shells are a potluck favorite! They taste and sound like they'd be more work than they are—especially if you use pre-made tomato sauce. It's also great because they're incredibly delicious. Isn't that all you could ask for?

Serves: 6

1 box jumbo pasta shells

Filling:
1 1/2 blocks of firm tofu
1 medium onion, diced
3-4 large cloves of garlic, minced
1/2 cup nutritional yeast
2   Tbsp olive oil
1 tsp lemon juice
salt and pepper to taste!
Optional/recommended:
small handful of pine nuts, chopped; a couple tsp each chopped fresh basil and chopped parsley

White Sauce:
1/2 cup (one stick) margarine
6   Tbsp flour
2-3 cup soymilk

2 cup tomato sauce (homemade or from a jar)

Preheat oven to 350 and grease a large casserole dish. Start boiling a large pot of salted water.

Begin by sautéing the onion and about three fourth of the garlic in your olive oil until soft. Reserve the rest of your garlic raw.

Meanwhile, start boiling your pasta shells according to the box (probably about 12 minutes).

Then, squeeze as much water as possible out of the tofu. Once you have done this, crumble it with your hands into a large mixing bowl. Smash it together with the cooked onions and garlic with their oil, and the rest of your filling ingredients (including the raw garlic). Add salt and pepper to taste. Don't be afraid to taste it at this point!

While the shells finish cooking, prepare your white sauce by melting the margarine in a saucepan over low-medium heat and adding the flour to make a paste. Once this is done, add the soymilk slowly, stirring constantly until you have a creamy, thick white sauce. Add salt to taste.

Once the shells are cooked, drain them and get out your filling, sauces, and casserole pan. Fill each shell with a large spoonful of filling, and place them in rows close together in the pan. Top each with a spoonful of white sauce, then a spoonful of tomato sauce. Bake at 350 for thirty minutes.

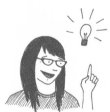

Ridiculously Useful Tip: After you drain the shells, you can put them back in the pot and cover with cold water. This will make them cool enough to handle so you can fill them. Scoop 'em out one at a time and shake the water off (gently!).

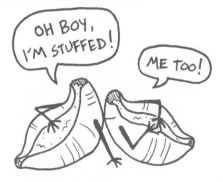

OH BOY, I'M STUFFED!

ME TOO!

Garlicky Mashed Sweet Potatoes with Kale

Among my circle of friends, this is considered pretty much the ultimate side to a meal of healthy comfort foods (which usually also involves barbecue tofu—try it!). Sweet potatoes make this just the right amount of sweet and savory, while the garlic gives it a healthy kick and the kale, well, kale is super healthy and green and great. I say it serves four, but let's get real, you could probably eat all of it yourself.

Serves: 4

2 large yams, about 4 cup chopped
3 big kale leaves, about 1 cup minced
3 cloves garlic, minced
1/4 cup soymilk
2 Tbsp margarine
1/4 tsp onion powder
salt to taste

Start boiling water in a large pot. Peel the yams and cut them into one inch pieces. Throw the pieces into the water once it boils, and cook for about fifteen minutes until they are tender and can be mashed with a fork.

In the meantime, mince your kale and garlic nice and small. When the yams are done cooking, drain and return them to your large pot. Throw in the kale, garlic and margarine, and start mashing with a potato masher or fork or something. Slowly add the soymilk and keep mashing 'til the whole thing is your preferred creamy consistency. Add onion powder and salt to taste.

Asparagus with Zingy Roasted Garlic Sauce

I hate to say something like "zingy", but you know—that's what this sauce is. Tons of garlic, tons of lemon juice. What else is there to say? The perfect accompaniment to steamed asparagus. Also great on lots of other veggies, but I think this makes an especially refreshing and satisfying pair.

Serves: 2-4

1 lb skinny asparagus stalks

Sauce:
ten large cloves garlic, about half a head of garlic
2 tsp olive oil
2   Tbsp lemon juice (from 1 1/2 to 2 lemons)
1   Tbsp additional olive oil
1   Tbsp soymilk
pinch of salt
pinch of pepper

Preheat your oven to 400.

Peel your garlic and toss with two tsp olive oil. Wrap it in a piece of tinfoil and put on a baking sheet or in an oven-safe pan to prevent garlic leakage from sullying your oven. Place into hot oven and roast for fifteen-18 minutes, until the garlic is very soft and mashable with a fork.

Meanwhile, wash and chop the tough ends off your asparagus. Place in a large shallow pan with a few Tbsp water, and steam, covered, over medium heat for about ten minutes. I like my asparagus "al dente", so I check for doneness by tasting a piece. You can taste a piece yourself and steam it 'til it's cooked how you like.

When the garlic is done roasting, take it out of the oven and open up the tinfoil packet on a cutting board. Smash the garlic with a fork until it is thoroughly mashed and pretty much a paste.

In a small bowl, add the mashed garlic to the rest of the sauce ingredients and whisk into a homogeneous mixture with your fork. Serve over asparagus and enjoy!

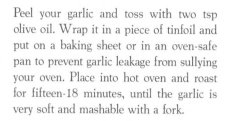

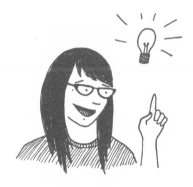

Ridiculously Useful Tip: This sauce is good on all kinds of vegetables, not just asparagus! Try it on anything roasted, like Brussels sprouts, potatoes, broccoli, or cauliflower.

Tasty Tangy Barbecue Sauce

It was not until adulthood that I started to like barbecue sauce. In fact, it wasn't until long after I became vegan that I thought it made a good addition to anything. So, ironic as it may or may not be, I always associate this with barbecue tofu, rather than a hamburger, or even a veggie burger. I guess what I'm saying is: slap it on some super-firm tofu and grill the hell out of it to see what I'm daydreaming about as I write this.

Makes: about 3 cups of sauce

2   Tbsp oil
1 medium onion, minced
2 cup ketchup
1/4 cup packed brown sugar
1/2 cup tomato paste
2   Tbsp molasses
2   Tbsp white vinegar
1/4 cup orange juice
1 tsp soy sauce
1 1/2 tsp liquid smoke
1/2 tsp paprika
1/4 tsp chili powder
1/4 tsp black pepper

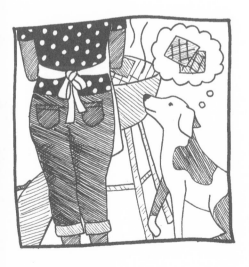

Sauté the onion in the oil until soft—about ten minutes. Add all remaining ingredients to your hot pan and simmer over low heat, stirring frequently, for about twenty minutes. Puree your sauce in a blender or food processor 'til smooth (no more onion bits!). It can be thinned with a little water if need be.

Slather it on anything that needs a tangy kick—like tofu—and you're good to go!

Three Bean Chili with Veggies

This is what you want to make if you have a touring band staying at your house, or a bunch of hungry roommates, or it's winter and you want to cook once and freeze the rest of your food in individually-sized portions and freeze it for the coming months. It's good and it'll fill you up!

Serves: 6

1 small onion (or half a large onion), diced
3 cloves garlic, minced
2 carrots, diced
2 medium zucchini, diced
1 cup corn (I use frozen)
2 (15oz.) cans kidney beans
1 (15oz.) can black beans
1 (15oz.) can garbanzo beans
1 (15oz.) can tomato sauce
1 cup TVP (see the ingredient primer for more on this)
1 1/2 cup vegetable broth, or water plus one bouillon cube
4   Tbsp olive oil
3   Tbsp nutritional yeast
Spices (this is fairly mild; you can use more to taste!):
1 tsp cumin
1 tsp paprika
1/4 tsp cayenne
1/4 tsp onion powder
1/4 tsp garlic powder
1/2 tsp salt

In a large pot, begin to cook the onion and garlic in olive oil. Next, add your diced carrots and zucchini. Sprinkle a little salt over the whole thing and mix together. Cover the pot and sauté the mixture over medium heat, stirring occasionally. Cook until all the vegetables are tender and just about cooked through, about ten minutes total.

Next add the beans (if they are canned, rinse first!) and the tomato sauce. Then add the TVP and vegetable broth and mix it all together. Starting to look like chili yet? A little bit?

Slowly add your spices, tasting as you go! You can add more cayenne if you like a spicier chili. Simmer over medium heat, covered, for about thirty minutes. In the last five or ten minutes of cooking, stir in the corn and nutritional yeast.

Serve with bread or rice and feed the masses!

Butternut Squash Macaroni

A play off mac and cheese that, once you taste it, you'll realize is all about that rich, roasted veggie flavor. Of course it's also got the requisite soymilk, margarine, and nutritional yeast, so best of both worlds!

Serves: 4

1 smallish (1 lb) butternut squash
2   Tbsp margarine
1/3 cup soymilk
1   Tbsp nutritional yeast
3/4 tsp salt
1/4 tsp onion powder
1/4 tsp garlic powder
1 pinch paprika
couple tsp olive oil
4 cup cooked macaroni, or pasta of your choice

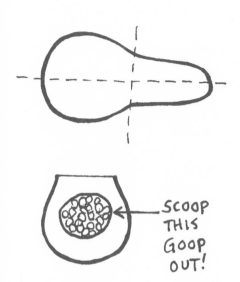

SCOOP THIS GOOP OUT!

Heat your oven to 425 and cut your butternut squash according to the diagram, like so:

Scoop the seeds out of the round bottom half. Coat the surfaces with olive oil, and place face-down in an oven-safe pan. Roast at 425 for about fourty five minutes, until the flesh is mashable with a fork.

Scoop the cooked flesh out of the skin and into a blender. Blend along with margarine and soymilk until it's all smooth and creamy.

Now move it into a saucepan and heat over medium heat as you mix in the seasonings. Add more salt and nutritional yeast to taste if you like.

Toss with your cooked pasta and enjoy!

Twice-Baked Shepard's Pie-tatoes

The name is kind of a mouthful—shepard's pie meets twice-baked potatoes and has a delicious baby with a crispy potato shell, savory filling, and fluffy mashatato topping? Did you get all that from the name? Because that's what it's trying to tell you. That and, "Make these now and invite a bunch of friends over for dinner because they will be delighted and impressed and it's not even that hard." Well, go on.

Serves: 4-8

4 russet potatoes, cleaned, dried and rubbed with a bit of oil
1 cup frozen mixed vegetables (I like the kind with carrots, peas, corn, and green beans)
1 cup fake meaty crumbles (for this I use the frozen Boca brand crumbles, but anything "beefy" will work)
1/2 cup (one stick) margarine
2 Tbsp flour
1/2 small onion, diced
2 cloves garlic, minced
3/4 cup vegetable broth (or bouillon plus water)
5 Tbsp soymilk
1 Tbsp nutritional yeast
salt and pepper to taste

Preheat oven to 400 while you clean and oil your potatoes. Once the oven is hot and your potatoes are ready to go, bake them whole for one hour, until the skin is crisp and the potato is easily pierced with a fork. Once they are done, set the potatoes on a wire cooling rack for at least fifteen minutes, until they start to cool enough to be handled.

Now turn your oven up to 450 in preparation for the second baking.

While your potatoes are in the oven baking, prepare your filling! Take half your margarine (1/4 cup), and heat over medium until it melts. Add in your diced onion and garlic and sauté until they begin to soften. Then, add your flour to the mixture and whisk until it is thoroughly combined and forms a paste. Next, stir in your vegetable broth. Keep over medium heat and keep stirring until the whole thing thickens and becomes creamy. Now you can add in your vegetables and meaty crumbles, and mix until they are all thoroughly coated. Add salt and pepper to taste and set aside until the potatoes are ready to be filled.

Now it's time to cut and prepare your potatoes. Use an oven mitt or towel to handle them, since they'll probably still be effing hot. Cut each in half lengthwise, according to the illustration. Each half should have a fairly wide, flat side to rest on. With a small spoon, scoop out most of the innards from each potato half, leaving about one eighth to one fourth in each shell. Place the shells on a baking sheet and return to the oven for a few minutes until they have gotten slightly more dry and crisp.

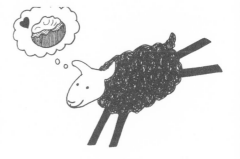

Meanwhile, prepare your mashed potato topping! Take about two thirds of the potato innards you've scooped out, and smash with a fork or mix with an electric mixer, along with the rest of your margarine, the soymilk, nutritional yeast, and salt to taste until fluffy and well-combined.

Take your potato shells out of the oven again and get ready to fill! Scoop a couple spoonfuls of the filling into each one, so they are full to just about the top of the shell (or a little less). Then, spread some of our mashed potato mixture over the top. Do this with each shell, and when they are all done, bake them in your 450 degree oven for about ten minutes, to heat the filling and slightly crisp the top.

The best!

Mango Sticky Rice

This is one of the best desserts ever. Or, being as it is made up of a grain and some fruit, I might even go so far as to say it could be one of the best breakfasts ever. The perfect ending to a Thai-style dinner, or any meal that could use a little sweetness—this is super easy to make and will thrill anyone you serve it to. Be sure to read the Ingredient Primer entry on sticky rice if you're not familiar with it, to make sure you get the right kind.

Serves: 8

1 1/2 cup Thai sticky rice
1 3/4 cup warm water
1 (14oz.) can coconut milk
3   Tbsp sugar
1/2 tsp salt
1 ripe, fresh mango, peeled and sliced

In a large glass or ceramic bowl, soak the rice with the warm water for at least twenty minutes. You can't skip this part, so don't even think about it!

Once the rice has been soaked, cover your bowl with a plate or other loose, lid-type thing, and stick it in the microwave. Yes, I said stick it in the microwave! Sticky rice is traditionally steamed, but the microwave makes quick work of cooking it without sacrifice. I was wary at first, but trust me on this one.

Microwave the rice, covered, for three minutes. Stir thoroughly, then put it back in for another three minutes. Stir again and check its cooking status. It probably needs another three to four more minutes to get all the way cooked, so pop it back in until it's done!

In the meantime, you can prepare your sauce. Heat the coconut milk in a large saucepan with the sugar and salt. Stir until everything is well combined and the sugar is dissolved.

Once the rice and sauce are both done, pour third fourth of the coconut sauce over the rice and stir. Let this sit, covered, for five to ten minutes.

Now you can plate your rice. Stick a generous helping of mango slices on top, and spoon a couple tablespoons of your reserved coconut sauce over the top of the whole thing. Serve hot!

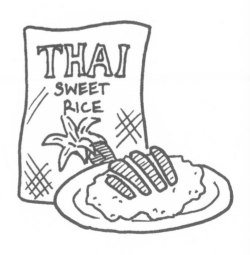

The Super Veggie Tahini Bowl

This is a simple and fast dinner that has it all: protein and texture from the tofu, nutrients from the veggies, filling from the grain, and creamy, zesty deliciousness from the tahini sauce. Whip it up on a weeknight and take your leftovers to work!

Serves: 4

1 1/4 cup (or one 10oz. package) couscous
2 cup water
1   Tbsp olive oil
1/2 tsp salt
1/2 tsp onion powder
1/2 tsp garlic powder

1 block extra firm tofu
Couple tablespoons oil, for frying
Couple squirts of Bragg's, or soy sauce

2 heads of broccoli, chopped
2 carrots, chopped
1/2 small onion, diced
5-6 big kale leaves, de-veined and chopped

For the sauce:
2 cloves garlic, finely minced
3   Tbsp tahini
2   Tbsp lemon juice (from one to two lemons)
2   Tbsp olive oil
3   Tbsp water
1/2 tsp onion powder
1/4 tsp salt

Boil water for your couscous. Add the olive oil, salt, and onion and garlic powder. Once the water comes to a rolling boil, turn off the heat and stir in the couscous. Let sit, covered, for at least five minutes.

Meanwhile, steam your veggies for a few minutes until they are tender. You can use a vegetable steamer for this if you have one, or if not, put a small amount of water in a large pan with the vegetables and cook them, covered, over medium-high heat until they start to soften. Put the kale in last, for just a minute or so, to avoid wilting the shit out of it.

Drain and slice your tofu into little cubes and get ready to fry it with the oil and a little Bragg's for flavor. The more health-conscious may not love this, but it's what makes it so damn good. I fry tofu in a nonstick pan over relatively high heat, making sure to turn each piece frequently to get each side of the cube evenly cooked and crispy.

Now you've got to prepare your tahini sauce. In a small bowl or cup, mix the oil into the tahini, then add the lemon juice and water to thin it out. You can use more or less water depending how thick you want your sauce, so add slowly for maximum control. Mix in the minced garlic and spices, and add more to taste if need be.

Now it's time to assemble your bowl! Layer some of the couscous, then veggies, then tofu. Scoop a generous serving of tahini sauce over the top of it all and mix it all up to enjoy!

Bacon(ish)

All the "facon"-type names were taken by name brand substitutes. So let's say it's bacon(ish). Which is kind of perfect. It's like the salty-savory-smoky meat, but kinder to our little pig friends and your health. Warning: you're gonna need a food processor for this one.

Makes: a whole bunch! Enough for a Sunday brunch full of friends.

1/2 cup cannellini beans
1/4 cup vital wheat gluten
1/4 cup bread crumbs
1 tsp canola oil
3 Tbsp soy sauce
2 Tbsp nutritional yeast
2 Tbsp maple syrup
1 Tbsp tomato paste
1 Tbsp liquid smoke
pinch of garlic powder
pinch of onion powder
oil for fry

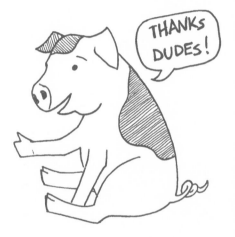

Preheat your oven to 375.

Process all ingredients in your food processor until they are a combined paste.

Roll a teaspoon or two at a time into little logs, then, with a bowl of water to keep your hands slightly wet, press down into a bacon(ish) shape very thin onto a parchment covered baking sheet.

Bake for ten minutes, then move to a cooling rack to let them firm up for a few minutes.

Heat your oil for frying in a wide pan and fry the "bacon" in batches for about thirty seconds on each side, to give it that nice crunch!

Lemon-Basil Orzo

Orzo is quick and easy and full of flavor. Reducing the vegetable broth concentrates its flavor and ensures that the dish isn't too watery, while the addition of fresh lemon juice and basil give it a pesto-like tang without the time and energy required to make full-on pesto. What more could you ask for?

Serves: 4

1 cup orzo, uncooked
1/2 cup vegetable broth
2-3 cloves garlic, minced
2 Tbsp margarine
2-3 Tbsp lemon juice
salt and pepper, to taste
handful or fresh basil, chopped
handful of pine nuts

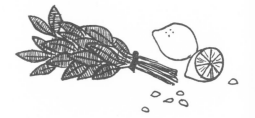

Cook the orzo as you would any pasta in boiling water for eight minutes or so, until it is al dente.

In a small saucepan, simmer the vegetable broth until it is reduced by half. Meanwhile, sauté the garlic in the margarine briefly, until it is just about cooked but maintains some fresh-garlic bite. Mix it in with the reduced broth.

When the orzo is cooked, drain it and toss with the broth/garlic mixture and lemon juice. Season it with salt and a generous amount of pepper, and top with your fresh basil and pine nuts!

"Throw Together" Salsas and Sides

This Black Bean and Corn Salad and the Mango Salsa on the next page are both what I call "throw together" recipes. That is, they don't have precise recipes, and can be eyeballed and taste-tested as you go for quick results without sacrificing anything in flavor or texture. There's no need for precision with something like this—it's all about how much of your ingredients you have on hand, and how you feel like tossing them together.

Black Bean and Corn Salad is a great side to tacos (or, hey, even a filling for tacos, if you like!), and Mango Salsa goes well with anything you want to give a tangy, sweet-savory kick. Neither of these are spicy at all, but you could add some minced peppers to either if that's how you roll.

Black Bean and Corn Salad

black beans, drained and rinsed if you use canned
fresh sweet corn, cut from the cob
red onion, minced
fresh lime juice
some diced tomato, if you like
salt to taste

Combine about two parts black beans to one part each corn and tomato, and one part minced onion. Season generously with lime juice and sprinkle with salt to taste.

Mango Salsa

1 large ripe mango, peeled, pitted, and diced
couple Tbsp red onion, diced small
one fourth to one half ripe avocado, diced
juice from one lime
salt to taste

Toss all ingredients together with lime juice and salt to taste.

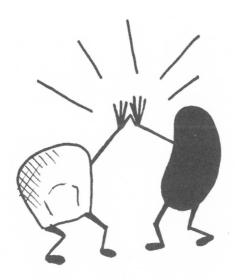

Basic Seitan

Seitan is a great savory, protein-laden meat substitute that is fun to make yourself and has the bonus of being able to be made in pretty much any amount you want! Once you get the hang of it, you can scale this recipe up or down easily. See the entry in the Ingredient Primer on seitan/vital wheat gluten for more information on what this stuff is about and where to shop for it.

1-2 cup vital wheat gluten
warm water, about equal to the amount of wheat gluten
Several   Tbsp soy sauce or Bragg's Liquid Aminos
Vegetable broth to fill a large stock pot
Spices of your choosing: nutritional yeast, onion and garlic powder, ground ginger, soy sauce, etc.

In a large mixing bowl, combine the wheat gluten and warm water and knead until it becomes a consistent texture. You can add in some spices of your choosing at this point— remember the seitan will take on flavor from the broth it is cooked in!

Run your seitan blob under cold water and knead until water runs clear. Alternately, you can complete this step by kneading it in a bowl of cold water, changing the water every minute or so until the water ceases to become milky from the seitan. If pieces start to fall off, don't worry, stick them back into the big chunk.

Meanwhile, prepare your stock pot with vegetable broth, as well as the soy sauce/ Bragg's and whatever else you may want to use to flavor your seitan.

Cut your seitan into about finger-seized pieces (they'll grow in the broth—creepy!) and boil in your covered pot for one hour. Hooray!

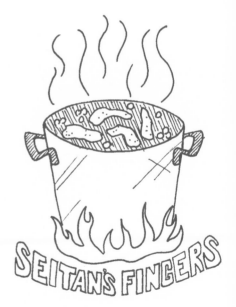

SEITAN'S FINGERS

Seitan Broccoli

All the charms of beef broccoli—assuming you're the type of person who's ever found beef broccoli charming—with none of the nasty cow parts. Serve it over rice for a healthy, tasty meal!

Serves: 4

1 cup prepared seitan (see pg 56 for recipe)
1 1/2 cup vegetable broth
1 lb (ish) broccoli
1 medium onion, diced
2   Tbsp cornstarch (or flour will do if you're in a pinch)
2   Tbsp soy sauce
1   Tbsp grated fresh ginger
pinch of onion and garlic powder

Mix the cornstarch (or flour), onion and garlic powder, and soy sauce into one cup of the broth.

Chop both your broccoli and seitan into bite sized chunks.

Heat a half cup of plain broth in a wok or pan and stir fry the seitan for five minutes or so 'til it is hot and starts to brown a bit on the outside. Now add the broccoli and onion and stir fry for another couple minutes until they are starting to become tender.

Add the ginger and your broth/spice mixture and cook until the veggies are done and everything is well coated in the sauce. Yes!

The Beaver Casablancas (Coconut Cream Pasta in a Cass-o-roll)

By Seth Kramer

Do you feel constant pressure to impress your housemates with your culinary skills, but can't think of anything to make aside from stir fry or marinara sauce pasta or even BBQ tofu and mashed potatoes, if you are feeling daring? That's where this came from, and it won, especially with a simple beet salad. And some garlic bread. And some wine.

Serves: about 4

1 lb penne pasta
1 can of coconut milk
1/2 cup margarine (1 stick or 1/4 of a tub of Earth Balance!)
~ 4 Tbsp flour
1 onion
2 cup sundried tomatoes
1 or 2 portabella mushroom tops (or any other equivalent type of mushroom, though portabellas work best!)
6 cloves of garlic
1 1/2 cup fresh basil
breadcrumbs
salt and pepper to taste
1/3 cup plain soymilk (optional)

Preheat your oven to 325.

Start out by cutting up and sautéing the onion, then add garlic, sundried tomatoes, mushrooms, and then basil for the last minute!

Boil pasta!

Put the margarine in a pan and melt on medium heat! Add the flour and mix until it turns into a paste! Turn the heat to low and mix in the coconut milk! It should turn thick and saucy in no time! If you are using the optional soymilk, add that in before the coconut milk to make it a bit more filling. Let it all heat until it is saucy!

Mix it all in the same pot you cooked it in, then transfer it into a casserole dish and cover it all with breadcrumbs!

Bake for about fifteen minutes. Take it out and let it cool, then eat the shit out of it!

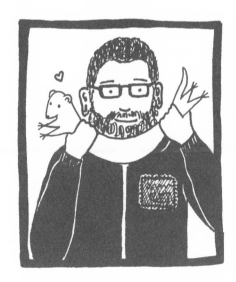

The Best Artichoke Dip

By Carolynn Webb

Based on a recipe I found years ago on the internet, this is a great dip for bread, crackers, veggies, or whatever you want. I like it as a sandwich spread. You'll need a food processor for this recipe!

1/2 cup raw almonds or if using blanched use 1/4 cup raw pin nuts
1/4 cup artichoke hearts (frozen or in the jar is fine, avoid the kind with a crazy marinade)
juice from 1 lemon
2-6 cloves garlic
1 Tbsp olive oil
1/4 tsp salt

*Blanched almonds are way more convenient!

If you use raw almonds you will need to remove the skin. If you want to keep it raw, place the almonds in a bowl, cover with water, and let soak in the fridge for a couple hours or overnight. Drain and squeeze the almond between your fingers and you can pop the almond out of the skin.

If you don't care about it being raw or are in a rush, pour boiling water over the almonds in a bowl. Let sit until it's cool enough to touch. Drain and squeeze the almonds.

Place almonds and pine nuts into a food processor and pulse until finely ground. Drain artichokes. Add garlic, artichokes, lemon juice, olive oil, and salt, and process until smooth. Scrape down side and adjust seasonings to taste. Add a little bit of water to get the consistency you want. Garnish with whole pine nuts.

Store in an airtight container in the fridge!

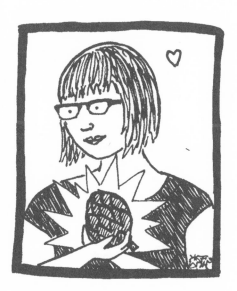

Lentil Soup

By Lorna Vetters

While not much on paper, including its lackluster name (though it's been referred to by my friend Gillian as "Salty Scottish") this soup has always been a standard in my family. It's quick and easy to make, cheap as hell, and delicious. But heads up: You're going to need a hand blender.

Serves: 4-6

Oil
1 medium onion (or half), chopped
2 carrots, chopped
2 cloves garlic, chopped (optional)
1 cup red lentils
6 cup water or vegetable broth
1   Tbsp sea salt (less if you're using salty broth)
pepper to taste

Lube up your soup pot with oil and sauté the onions. While they're cooking, chop the carrots and add them to the pot. Cook the onions until they're soft/translucent (don't worry about the carrots—they're just along for the ride). Add the garlic and cook a couple more minutes.

Add the lentils and water or broth, and bring up to a boil. Cover, reduce to a simmer, and cook for about thirty minutes, until the lentils are broken up and the carrots are soft enough to cut with the back of a knife.

Blend until smooth (or if you're like my mum in the '70s, you'll scrape it through a sieve with a wooden spoon) and salt it. Most important, and often screwed up, are the texture and saltiness of this soup. It's

not split pea soup; it should be fairly thin. And salt is a flavour enhancer, so don't be shy about adding the proper amount (unless you use broth)—I measured it for the first time for you!

Suggestion: Serve with fresh bread and some big IPAs, and surround yourselves with cats and some silly pugs.

Ed. Note: The extra "u"s in some of these words are all "sic." They remain to honour Lorna's Canadian roots!

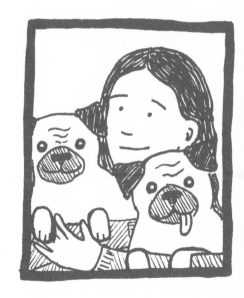

Creamy Cheese Sauce

By Tamar Shirinian

This recipe can be used for anything that requires a cheese sauce: nachos, chili cheese fries, mac and cheese, poured over broccoli, etc. Way better than any gross thing that's not vegan or comes in a box.

This makes enough for a large casserole. But you can make less by decreasing the amounts, or make a lot and store for use more than once!

3/4 cup canola oil
1 cup flour
5 cup of boiling water
1 3/4 cup nutritional yeast flakes
3 cloves of garlic (minced or crushed)
1 tsp turmeric powder
2   Tbsp soy sauce
salt and pepper to taste

Pour the oil into a sauce pan on medium heat, add flour bit by bit, and stir until creamy and thickening.

Add the boiling water. The mixture will get thick quite quickly. Lower heat.

Add garlic, nutritional yeast flakes, turmeric powder, soy sauce, salt and pepper. Stir well for five minutes.

cheese sauce rules!

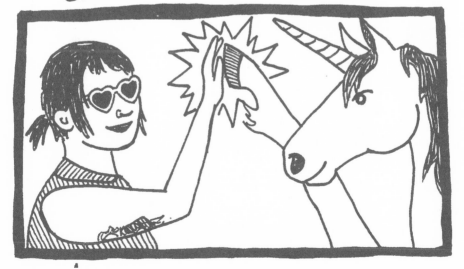

The Tofu Benedict

By Gina Fun Punx Giarrusso

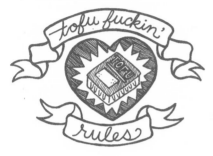

I should preface this recipe saying that Ashley does not like the idea of a benedict, whether it's vegan or not. She has not tried this recipe, but knows how much others like it. The benedict at Fellini in Berkeley, Ca was the best on the west coast—I've tried them all—so now that Fellini is closed, we'll all have to make do with this recipe.

Serves: 2

For the tofu scramble:
1 (14oz.) container of firm tofu
3 large cloves of garlic
1/2 tsp turmeric
1 tsp curry powder
1 Tbsp nutritional yeast
Olive oil (not sure of measurements, but everyone should have a whole bottle on hand all the time, anyway. While hitchhiking around Europe for four months, I had a ten oz. bottle of olive oil in my bag at all times, no joke. It will save some otherwise gross vegan food! [Yes, I'm Italian])

For the "hollandaise sauce":
1/2 tub (6oz.) "Toffuti" brand sour cream (sorry for the brand name!)
1 Tbsp margarine (I use Earth Balance)
1 Tbsp spicy yellow mustard (or regular mustard)
2 to 3 Tbsp lemon juice
1 Tbsp nutritional yeast

Additional Ingredients:
2 English muffins
4 slices of "Yves" (once again sorry for the brand name) Canadian bacon

First make a tofu scramble to substitute the eggs in the benedict. You can always add extra whatever-you-want to a tofu scramble (onions, bell pepper, whatever), but here's how to make a very basic scramble: Press or finely cut the garlic into a pan. Douse the garlic in oil (until garlic is fully submerged in oil) and sauté on high until the oil is boiling, then reduce heat to low. Continue to sauté for about a minute and add in the block of tofu. Smash it all up with a potato masher or the back side of a fork until the tofu is crumbly.

Add turmeric, curry powder, nutritional yeast, and salt and pepper to taste. Cook until your tofu is a nice mushy texture. If it's watery, continue to cook until the tofu-water (yuck!) has cooked off. If it's not nice and mushy, put to the side on low heat to keep warm.

Now you're ready to make the "hollandaise" sauce! If you follow this recipe and try the sauce on its own, it will be STRONG. Don't be alarmed. After you apply it to the tofu, it will be the best.

Put all sauce ingredients into a bowl and microwave them for about 40 seconds. Mix together with a spoon until creamy.

Time to construct the benedict of your dreams!

Toast your English muffins. Pan cook Canadian bacon until it's how you like your bacon. Place cooked Canadian bacon on top of toasted English muffins.

Use some type of rounded spoon (an ice cream scooper even) to scoop one quarter of your tofu portion per each muffin.

Douse the tofu/muffin creation with your "hollandaise" sauce and top with a sprinkle of pepper.

I serve my Tofu benedict with some delicious potatoes—home fries, hash browns, etc. Enjoy! Added bonus: If you double the recipe and keep the leftovers in the fridge, you can throw everything into a tortilla for a delicious vegan breakfast "burrito"!

This recipe endorsed by Fun and Punx.

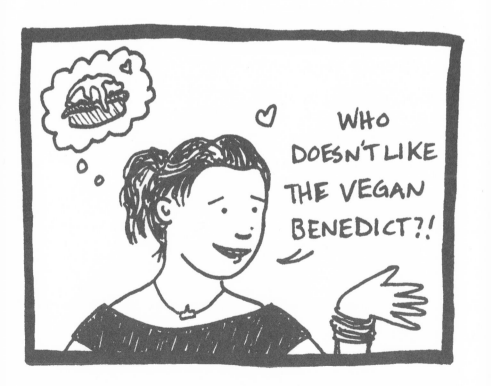

Camelia's Tortillas De Harina (Flour Tortillas)

By Camelia Rivera (with Mariana Palafox)

The first time I met Camelia, she taught me to make these tortillas. I was blown away by how amazingly delicious they are and how effortless she made them look. I practiced a few times and got the technique down, but was having a hard time getting the measurements exactly right. Fortunately, she wrote down this recipe to share. –A

Makes: 12

4 cup flour—La Pina brand is great, but any flour will do
1 tsp salt
1 cup soft vegetable shortening, like Crisco
2 cup boiling water

In a large bowl, mix together the flour and salt. Then mix in the shortening. Add boiling water a little at a time and mix with a large spoon. When it becomes too thick, start kneading the dough with your hands. Knead for a couple minutes and then let sit for two minutes before kneading again. Repeat two more times, and let sit for five minutes.

After the dough has rested for five minutes, form it into small, round balls. Roll with a rolling pin until they're very thin and as round as you can make them.

Cook on a skillet over medium-high heat. First, cook one side for just a few seconds. When you lift it up, it will look like it's just begun to cook, with parts of it lighter white, but no browning happening yet.

Flip it over and cook on the other side for a few more seconds. Now go ahead and flip it over—you'll have two more flips to do!

On the next flip, your tortilla will start to puff up with air. This is great, because it means the inside is cooking and all is well. Turn it over when the underside has got a little bit of color in some spots.

This will be your final flip. The tortilla will puff up like crazy now, and it's your job to (carefully!) poke it down and burst the bubbles as they come up with your hand covered by a clean cloth. When it's bubbled for a minute and the underside has some slight browning, your tortilla is done!

Repeat with the others and serve warm.

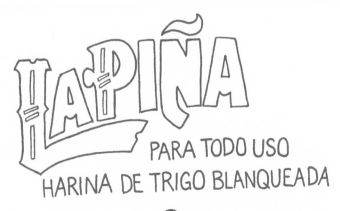

Camelia's Salsa

By Camelia Rivera (with Mariana Palafox)

Nothing more perfect to go with the wonderful tortillas you just made than some simple, fresh salsa!

4 large vine ripened tomatoes
3 or 4 cloves of garlic
3 or 4 serrano peppers
1 small yellow onion

Roast all the ingredients on the grill or in a lightly oiled cast iron pan—this will give the salsa a smoky flavor. After getting the veggies nice and roasted peel the skin off the tomatoes and give everything a rough chop in the blender. Add salt to taste. For an authentic flavor use a stone molcajete and mash all the ingredients together.

Debbie's Apple Spice Cake

By Debbie Nguyen

This was Debbie's first foray into vegan baking and, despite her nervousness, the cake was a huge hit at our dinner party! Seriously, it's enough to convert any nonbeliever. Especially perfect for holiday meals, but you don't have to wait for fall to roll around—make it whenever! —A

Serves: 12

1 1/2 plus 1/4 cup sugar, divided
1 1/2 cup flour
1/2 cup (one stick) margarine, softened
1 1/2 tsp baking powder
1 tsp vanilla
1/4 tsp salt
3/4 cup Tofutti vegan cream cheese, softened
2 tsp cinnamon
2 eggs' worth of egg-replacer (Debbie uses Ener-G brand)
3 cup chopped, peeled apples

Preheat your oven to 350.

Beat the cup and a half of sugar, margarine, vanilla and vegan cream cheese with an electric mixer until well-blended, then add in egg-replacer and beat well.

In a separate bowl, whisk together dry ingredients. Once mixed, add these to the wet mixture and beat together gently.

Combine your remaining half cup sugar and the cinnamon. Toss two Tbsp of this mixture with the chopped apples in a bowl, then stir the apple mixture into your cake batter.

Pour the batter into a greased 8" springform pan and sprinkle the rest of your sugar-cinnamon mixture over the top. Bake for one hour and fifteen minutes, or until the cake starts to pull away from the sides of the pan. Cool completely on a wire rack before serving!

The Best Basil Pesto

By Carolynn Webb

Pesto is an idiosyncratic dish. There are a million ways of combining the same basic ingredients. I like the pesto I grew up with—a brightly flavored vegan-by-default dish with lots of lemon and garlic. But since taste is subjective and this is so easy to make, you can easily adjust this recipe to fit your personal taste. It's lovely on pasta, on a sandwich, on grilled veggies, or anything.

Makes: 2/3 cup

1/3 cup pine nuts
2 cup packed fresh basil leaves
3 large cloves of garlic
2 Tbsp olive oil
juice from one lemon, about 2 Tbsp
Salt to taste

Wash the basil and take the leaves off the stems.

Put the pine nuts in your food processor* and pulse until finely ground.

Next, place basil, peeled garlic, lemon juice, salt, and olive oil into the food processor. Process until smooth, stopping occasionally to scrape down the sides. If the pesto seems thick, add a little water or an extra dash of olive oil.

Taste it and adjust as you see fit!

Before serving with pasta, thin out the sauce with some of the pasta water for the best consistency.

*You can also use a blender for this recipe. It's more of a pain but totally doable. Follow the directions above, but add a little more oil or water while blending. You're going to have to scrape down the blender a bunch of times, but it'll come together!

The Brown Justin

By Justin Rowe

Here's a clever way to use that box of fruit from Washington your grandmother sends you every Xmas: it's the Brown Justin!

Serves: 8

4 apples, peeled and quartered
4 pears, peeled and quartered
heaping 1/2 tsp ground cinnamon
1/2 tsp allspice
3 Tbsp brown sugar
1 tsp vanilla extract
2 Tbsp margarine, cut into little pieces
1/4 cup water

Preheat your oven to 325.

Place the apple and pear chunks into a roasting dish so that all pieces are touching and pour in the fourth cup water. Sprinkle cinnamon, allspice and brown sugar over all apples and pears, then drizzle with vanilla extract. Put one small piece of margarine on each piece of fruit. Cute!

Bake for thirty minutes or until golden brown.

Serve with a scoop of vanilla soy ice cream!

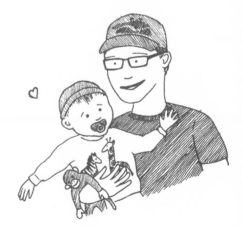

Debbie's Veggie Udon

By Debbie Nguyen

This recipe is delicious with its savory shiitake, and the kombu adds yummy umami flavor. You are advised to add as much mirin as you like; it only makes the broth better! It takes a little bit of prep time, but is so satisfying and worth it.

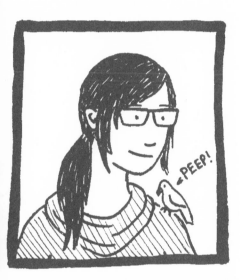

5-6 cup water
1 or 2 slices of kombu seaweed
1 cup dried, sliced shiitake mushrooms
1 cup fresh sliced shiitake mushrooms
2 large carrots, chopped
4 medium-sized red radishes, sliced thin
2 shallots or 1 small sweet yellow onion
1 package of ready to go udon noodles (in the refrigerated section)
2-3 stalks of sliced green onions
shoyu to taste
1 cup mirin
2-4 Tbsp of sesame oil
2-4 Tbsp of dried wakame seaweed
salt to taste
sugar to taste

Sauté your shallots or onion with the sesame oil in a stockpot until translucent and aromatic. Now fill the stockpot with water, and add kombu and dried shiitake. Bring to a boil, then simmer for ten-fifteen minutes.

Add the fresh shiitake, shoyu, mirin, salt, and sugar (remember to keep tasting!) and simmer for five minutes.

Now add the udon, carrots, radishes, green onions, and simmer for five more minutes. Serve with soaked wakame on the side!

Cashew Bell Pepper Cheese

By Tiffany & Sylvee Esquivel

A non-dairy, non-soy "cheesy" alternative. This cheese is amazing on pizza, pasta dishes, and as a spread!

4   Tbsp corn oil
1 red or orange bell pepper
2 tsp sea salt
½ cup raw cashews
½ onion, diced
5 cloves of garlic
2 cup water
2   Tbsp tapioca starch
2   Tbsp crushed oregano
2 tsp smoked paprika
½ of a lime, juiced

Preheat oven to 400 degrees. Brush 1 Tbsp corn oil over the bell pepper and bake for 35 minutes. Add the sea salt and cashews for the last fifteen minutes. In a sauce pan, cook your onion and garlic in two cups of water for three minutes. Remove the baked bell pepper and cashews from the oven and blend them with the cooked onions, garlic, and all remaining ingredients.

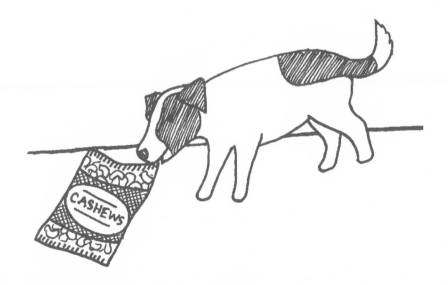

Moussaka

By Tiffany & Sylvee Esquivel

Moussaka is a baked eggplant-potato dish from Greece and the Middle East. It is comprised of eggplant and potatoes with layers of "cheese" and traditional Béchamel sauce.

3 eggplants, peeled and cut lengthwise into 1/2 thick slices
2 potatoes, peeled and cut thinly into ovals
1/4 cup olive oil
1 Tbsp butter
1 pound oyster mushrooms, chopped
2 onions, chopped
1 clove garlic, minced
1/4 tsp ground cinnamon
1/4 tsp ground nutmeg
1/2 tsp oregano
2 Tbsp dried parsley
2 tomatoes, cut and seeded
1/2 cup red wine
3 Tbsp potato starch
1 Tbsp non-dairy milk
salt and pepper to taste

For the "cheese:"
1 brick of extra firm tofu
3 Tbsp potato starch
1 Tbsp non-dairy milk
1 tsp ground nutmeg

For the Béchamel sauce:
4 cup non-dairy milk
1/2 cup vegan "butter"
6 Tbsp unbleached all purpose flour
salt
pepper

Preheat your oven to 350 degrees.

Lay the slices of eggplant on paper towels, sprinkle lightly with salt and set aside for thirty minutes to draw out the moisture. Quickly fry the eggplant in olive oil over high heat until browned. Set aside on paper towels to soak up excess oil.

Melt butter in a large skillet over medium heat, add the mushroom, onions, garlic, salt, and pepper to taste. After the mushrooms have browned, sprinkle in the cinnamon, nutmeg, oregano, and parsley. Pour in the tomatoes and wine and mix well. Simmer for twenty minutes. Allow to cool, and then beat in three Tbsp. potato starch and "milk."

In a large bowl, crumble together the tofu, potato starch, milk, and nutmeg to make a cheesy middle.

To make the béchamel sauce, begin by scalding the milk in a saucepan. Melt the butter in a large skillet over medium heat. Whisk in flour until smooth. Lower heat; gradually pour in the hot milk, whisking constantly until it thickens. Season with salt and pepper and remove from heat. It should stay white in color.

Arrange a layer of potatoes then a layer of eggplant in a greased 9x13 inch baking dish. Cover eggplant with all of the mushroom mixture, and then sprinkle half of cheese mixture over the mushroom. Cover with remaining eggplant, and sprinkle remaining cheese over. Pour the béchamel sauce over the top, and sprinkle with the nutmeg.

Bake for one hour.

Tzatziki

By Tiffany & Sylvee Esquivel

This creamy yogurt-salad is super versatile and can be used to accompany crisp vegetables, pita triangles, falafels, etc.
3 cup non-dairy yogurt
1 cucumber, peeled, seeded, and chopped
2 garlic cloves, finely minced
3 Tbsp fresh dill
1/4 cup olive oil
1/4 cup chopped fresh mint
Juice of 1/2 lemon
Parsley for garnish
salt
pepper

Use your hands to drain any liquid out of cucumbers.

In a large bowl mix yogurt, cucumber, garlic, fresh dill, oil, mint, lemon juice, salt and pepper.

Cover and rest in refrigerator for two hours. Garnish when chilled completely.

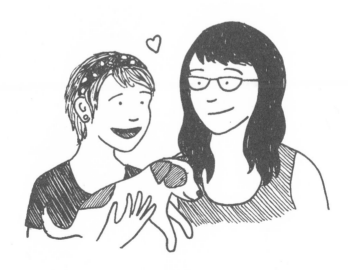

Mole Verde

By Tiffany & Sylvee Esquivel

Mole is a flavorful sauce popularly prepared in parts of Southern Mexico such as Oaxaca. Moles are bursting with amazing flavors and come in different varieties. Other popular moles include mole amarillo, mole rojo, and mole negro.

1 cup pumpkin seeds
fifteen medium six tomatoes, whole
1 cup spinach or other greens
1 onion, diced
3 serano peppers
4 jalapeños
Pinch of salt
6 cloves of garlic

Toast the pumpkin seeds over medium heat. Shake the pan around every five seconds to avoid burning the seeds. Set aside to cool when all of the seeds have toasted evenly.

Bring a large pot of water to a boil. Add all ingredients—except pumpkin seeds—to the pot and allow to stew for thirty minutes.

Drain water from pot, reserving about four cups of liquid.

Place reserved water, stewed ingredients, and toasted pumpkin seeds into blender and blend until extremely smooth.

"Karma" Sprinkles

A substitute for parmesan cheese; you can use it in the same situations, but don't expect it to taste the same. I'm not sure if the name refers to the good karma you'll have for not eating real cheese, or the bad karma I'll have for ripping off a similarly-named, very expensive product that I like to eat but don't like to pay for. Wait a second, CIY (that's cooking-it-yourself) is never bad karma!

Makes: About 3/4 cup of sprinkles

1/2 cup chopped raw walnuts
1/2 cup nutritional yeast
1/2 tsp salt

Find some way to crush the shit out of the walnuts. You could use a food processor if you have one, or do it old school style with a mortar and pestle (that would rule), or find an even more crafty DIY (ahem, I mean CIY) way to do it, like using a hammer, or the bottom of a small jar, or some kind of handle of something. Whatever.

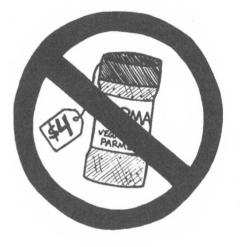

Once the walnuts are sufficiently pulverized, mix in the salt and nutritional yeast.

Store in an airtight container in the fridge for best results.

Spanish Rice

This is a recipe adapted from my mom's, which would be vegan except for all the ground beef in it. But who'd miss that anyway? If you're dead-set on the meaty texture you could throw in some TVP, but really, it doesn't need it. Stick it in burritos or eat it by itself!

Serves: 4-6

1 medium onion, diced
1/2 to 1 green bell pepper, seeded and chopped
2 cup rice, uncooked
2 cup water
1C tomato sauce
1/2 tsp salt
1/2 tsp onion powder
1/2 tsp garlic powder
1/4 tsp chili powder
olive oil (a couple Tbsp)

In a large pan over medium heat, sauté the onion and bell pepper in oil until almost soft.

Add the tomato sauce, then the rice, water and spices, and stir together.

Cover with a lid and simmer over low-medium heat until the rice is cooked, about twenty-twenty five minutes if you're using white rice. Stir occasionally so it doesn't stick. No one wants rice stuck all over the bottom of their pan, right? Right.

As always, spice to your preferences. Add more chili powder if you like some extra kick!

Zucchini Bread

Zucchini bread is one of those foods that sounds to the uninitiated unlike it tastes. While it does contain a whole bunch of fresh zucchini, it is very sweet and delicious, and decidedly not vegetable-y. It's rich and sweet and well-spiced, and I promise you will love it. Bonus: You can justify eating it for breakfast, since it's got such a high veggie-and-fruit content!

Makes: 2 loaves

1 cup canola oil
1 large banana, mashed
2 cup sugar
2 cup grated zucchini
3/4 of a small (8oz.) can of crushed pineapple
1 Tbsp vanilla
3 cup flour
1 Tbsp cinnamon
1 tsp baking soda
1 tsp baking powder
1 tsp salt
1/2 cup chopped walnuts
1/2 cup raisins (optional)

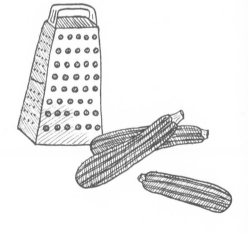

Preheat your oven to 325.

Beat together the banana, sugar and oil. Drain your pineapple very well, and add that and the grated zucchini and vanilla to the wet mixture. Mix together dry ingredients (not including nuts or raisins), and then stir slowly into wet to combine. Fold in nuts and raisins last.

Pour batter into two greased loaf pans and bake for about one hour and ten minutes (you can start checking around 50 minutes for doneness).

Dirty Rice to Feed the Masses

This is one of those dishes to make if you've got a touring band staying at your house and need a meal that's filling and easy to make a lot of. It's mostly a "pantry dish" that can be made with stuff you have on hand. Score!

Serves: Tons! Or 2-4 if you're extremely hungry.

4 cup rice, cooked in…
5 cup veggie broth
1 large onion, diced
garlic (like 5 cloves), minced
2 bell peppers, seeded and cut into slices
1 can black beans
1 can kidney beans
3/4 cup TVP, soaked in about 1/2 cup hot water to soften
1 1/4 cup tomato sauce
1/2 tsp thyme
1/2 tsp garlic powder
splash of soy sauce or Bragg's
pinch of nutritional yeast
olive oil, for sautéing
salt and pepper to taste

Start by chopping all your veggies and starting your rice and vegetable broth in a rice cooker or large pot. Heat up a little bit of oil in a large pan like a wok, and sauté together the onion, garlic, and bell pepper until they are cooked to your liking.

Appreciate the smell your kitchen's got going on right about now.

Next, add into your veggie mixture the TVP, along with all the beans and the tomato sauce. Mix in your seasonings (remember to taste!), and keep stirring until it's thoroughly mixed and hot.

Once the rice and the "dirty" slop are both done, mix them together and feed everyone!

Cucumber Salad

This cucumber salad is a Thai-style side that makes a great accompaniment to lots of different dishes, including anything fried. It's got a great, bright flavor, and serving it straight from the fridge makes it extra refreshing, in addition to giving all the flavors lots of time and space to mingle (if you know what I mean).

Serves: 2-4

1 large cucumber
¼ to ½ small red onion (depending how much onion you like)
1 small carrot, grated
5 Tbsp rice vinegar
1 Tbsp sugar
2 Tbsp warm water
½ tsp salt

Cut your cucumber in half long-ways, then into slices about one fourth inch thick. Scoop out the seeds from the middle, especially if your cucumber has lots! Slice the onion into very thin pieces, about one inch long, and grate your carrot. Toss all the veggies together in a big bowl.

Now prepare your dressing! First, stir the sugar and salt into the warm water to dissolve. Then, add in your vinegar and stir to combine. Pour the dressing over the salad and toss together until well-mixed.

Cover your bowl and stick the salad in the refrigerator for half an hour to let the flavors soak in and make sure it's nice and cold for serving. Serve as soon as it's done chillin'!

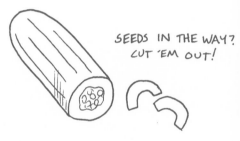

SEEDS IN THE WAY? CUT 'EM OUT!

(Sweeter Than) Honey

This recipe was stumbled upon when my baking partner Carolynn and I were trying to get the ratios and seasonings right to make a simple syrup for our baklava. Turns out, with the lemon and cardamom to give it a bit of a floral taste, and plenty of sugar to sweeten and thicken it up, it makes a fabulous substitute for honey!

As you can see from the ingredients list, it's almost pure sugar—but it's meant to be used sparingly! A little in your tea or on a peanut butter sandwich and you're golden!

Makes: about 1 ½ cups

1 3/4 cup sugar
¾ cup water
1 Tbsp lemon juice
ten peppercorns
4 whole cardamom seeds

Combine all ingredients in a saucepan and bring to a full boil. Keep stirring as your syrup heats up to make sure all the sugar dissolves. Once sugar is dissolved and the mixture has come to a boil, turn the heat off. Pour the syrup into a receptacle to cool. Once cooled, pick the peppercorns and cardamom seeds out and enjoy!

This non-honey stores well in the fridge!

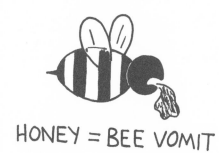

HONEY = BEE VOMIT

Potato Salad

I have to admit, I was a potato salad hater. I tried it as a kid, realized how gross mayo was to me, and never got over it. That is, until the garlic aioli in this recipe came into my life. I'm sorry to ask for a name brand product, as I know it may be hard or impossible for some of y'all to get your hands on. But I encourage you to try if you can, and fear not if you can't—check out the ridiculously useful tip below.

Serves: 4

8-ten medium sized red potatoes
1 large or 2 small carrots
large handful of black olives, sliced
1/3 cup red onion, sliced
For the sauce:
¾ cup Wildwood Garlic Aioli*
1 Tbsp olive oil
2 Tbsp lemon juice (about one lemon's worth)
½ tsp dried dill
salt and pepper to taste

Chop your vegetables! Cut potatoes into bite-sized cubes, and slice carrots and onion super thin. Meanwhile, start some water boiling to cook your potatoes.

Boil until potato chunks are tender and pierceable with a fork—about ten minutes. Once cooked, drain the potatoes and rinse with cold water to start them cooling off. Transfer to a large mixing bowl and stick 'em in the fridge until they start to get cold, at least fifteen minutes.

While the potatoes chill out, make your sauce by whisking together all the ingredients.

Once the potatoes are cool and the sauce is made, toss everything together and stir until coated thoroughly. Eat now or store in the fridge!

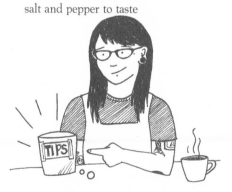

*Ridiculously useful tip: If you can't get your hands on the Wildwood aioli, but do have access to some other vegan mayo-type thing (whether it's store-bought, like Vegenaise, or homemade), try adding a small clove of garlic crushed or finely minced to the sauce part of this salad.

Sweet Little Corn Cakes

Corn "cakes" is somewhat of a misnomer as this recipe produces a moist spoonbread. I first fell in love with a similar dish as a kid eating at the admittedly inauthentic "Mexican" chain El Torito, which my family frequented for years. Years later, I was delighted to find I could modify it easily into a tasty vegan treat! It's sweet, rich, and extremely delicious; perfect as a dessert for a Southern or Mexican inspired dinner. Scoop it with an ice cream scoop and eat it with a spoon—how much more fun could it be?

Serves: 4-6

1/2 cup margarine
1/3 cup plus 1 Tbsp masa de harina
1/4 cup warm water
1/3 cup sugar
1/4 cup cornmeal
1/4 tsp salt
1/2 tsp baking powder
2 Tbsp soymilk
1 1/4 cup yellow corn kernels (I use frozen)

Preheat your oven to 350.

In a mixing bowl, cream your margarine with an electric mixer until it starts to get light and fluffy. Then, beat in the masa along with the water.

Coarsely chop the corn so that the kernels are broken up, but still chunky. This will add texture to your finished corn cakes! Once chopped, stir into the margarine/masa mixture.

Whisk together the sugar, cornmeal, salt, and baking powder, then stir into the wet mixture along with the soymilk.

Once everything is thoroughly combined, pour your batter into an ungreased pie tin, or 8"x8" baking pan and smooth the top. Place this pan into a larger baking or casserole dish with a half inch or so of water in it. This will ensure even cooking

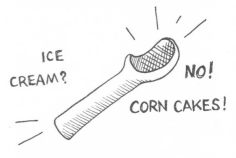

and help your corn cake to retain moisture in the oven while it bakes.

Stick the whole thing in the oven and bake at 350 for about 50 minutes. Allow it to cool for at least ten minutes after you take it out, and then scoop with an ice cream scoop or large spoon into delicious little domes (or piles, depending on whether or not you have an ice cream scoop and how much you care). Dig in!

Caramelized Roasted Carrots

These sweet roasted carrots are a perfect side dish for a holiday meal. Super easy and with almost no prep-time, they are guaranteed to delight even the staunchest vegetable-hater at your table.

Serves: 2-4

4 large carrots, peeled
3 Tbsp vegan margarine
2 Tbsp brown sugar
1/4 tsp salt

Preheat your oven to 400.

Slice carrots in half longways (kids you know may say "hotdog style", which is descriptive, and also, gross), and then into about one inch chunks.

Melt together the margarine and sugar, and add salt.

Line a casserole dish with aluminum foil or parchment and stick the carrots in it. Pour the margarine/sugar sauce over them, and cover it all with more foil.

Bake for twenty minutes, then give it a good stir and remove the foil. Bake for another fifteen minutes or so until the carrots are tender and the sauce is nice and caramelized on them.

Savory Maple Glazed Baked Tofu

This baked tofu is the perfect balance of savory and sweet, as well as having an awesome, chewy texture! Goes great with creamy mac and cheese or potatoes and a bright salad for a savory-sweet treat, and could nicely offset something spicy too, I suspect.

Serves: 4-6

16oz. super firm tofu, drained well
1/4 cup Braggs liquid aminos
2 Tbsp orange juice
4 cloves garlic, thinly sliced
1/2 cup maple syrup, divided

Start by slicing your tofu into sheets one fourth to one half inch thick. Mix together your Braggs and orange juice, and the garlic slices, and pour over the tofu. Let it marinate one hour so it'll soak up all the sweet and savory flavors.

Meanwhile, preheat your oven to 375 and line a casserole pan with aluminum foil or parchment.

Once your tofu slices are ready, put 'em down in a single layer along the bottom of the casserole pan. Place the garlic slices in the marinade with Braggs on top of them. Reserve and set aside the remaining marinade. Drizzle two Tbsp of the maple syrup over the tofu and put the pan into the oven, uncovered. Bake for fifteen minutes, then flip the pieces over and baste with two Tbsp more maple syrup. Bake for another fifteen minutes on this side before the final step.

While your tofu begins to bake, put your left over marinade into a small pan and add in your remaining maple syrup (should be a fourth cup). Reduce over low-medium heat for about five minutes, stirring occasionally until it is thickened and no longer super liquidy.

Finally, remove your tofu from the oven and flip it over one last time. Drizzle over each piece as much of your maple-marinade reduction as you desire. If you have some left over, that's okay. It's got a fairly strong flavor, and you can spread a little more on when your tofu is all done.

Stick it back in the oven and bake for another twenty five minutes or so, until the tofu has a chewy texture and a dark, caramelized-looking outside.

Serve it with the now-roasted garlic slices as a garnish bursting with flavor.

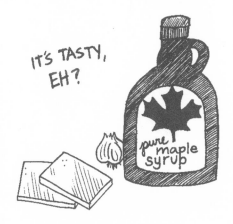

IT'S TASTY, EH?

pure maple syrup

Overnight Oatmeal

A unique breakfast treat, especially during the summertime when its cool, creamy consistency helps to fill you up without feeling too heavy. You prepare it the night before, too, so if you roll out of bed with, say, fifteen minutes before you need to leave the house, you can just scarf it down and be on your way. It's also supremely customizable.

Serves: 2

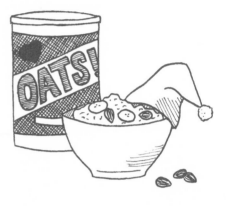

3/4 cup uncooked oats (not instant)
3/4 cup soymilk or nondairy milk of your choice (I like vanilla!)
1 (6oz.) container of nondairy yogurt, in your choice of flavor
1/2 banana, sliced thin
a couple tsp of brown sugar, optional
any other fruit, nuts, or granola you may like to top it with

Mix together your oats, soymilk, yogurt and banana slices in a bowl*. Cover and refrigerate overnight. In the morning, stir in brown sugar to taste, and top with any crunchy goodness that sounds appealing to you. Enjoy with a friend!

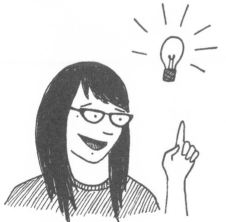

*Ridiculously useful tip: At this point you can also add any type of dried fruit you like (I like dried cranberries), and it will sort of rehydrate overnight as it absorbs some of the liquid. If that sounds good to you, go for it!

Pear Salad with Raspberry-Lemon Dressing

This salad's got a sweet-tart thing going on in a supremely satisfying way. I like to make it up to brighten up a fall or winter meal—conveniently also when pears are at their best, and use frozen raspberries, which are at their best all year round.

Serves: 2-4

3-4 cup spring mix (a few big handfuls)
1 small ripe pear, sliced thin
1/3 cup walnuts or pecans, chopped

Dressing:
2 Tbsp lemon juice (from one lemon)
1 1/2 tsp olive oil
1 tsp agave nectar
5 or so raspberries, smashed
salt and pepper to taste

Put your salad ingredients into a big bowl. Stick all the stuff to make the dressing in a small bowl or a glass, and whisk together with a fork to get a homogenous consistency. Add a tiny bit of salt and pepper—you can always sprinkle your salad with some more once it's assembled, if you want.

Pour the dressing over your salad and toss to evenly coat!

Nachos Your Way

God, what a good idea nachos are. A big pile of deliciousness, customizable in ingredients, proportions and size. Excellent for sharing with tons of friends. This recipe makes use of a couple others in this book, and beyond that, you're in complete control! Savor that power. And the nachos, too.

Serves: Whoever you've invited to your nacho party—make enough for just you or a whole crew!

You'll need:

Cashew Bell Pepper Cheese (recipe on pg. 66)
or
Creamy Cheese Sauce (recipe on pg. 57)
Don't-fuck-it-up Guacamole (recipe on pg. 16)
tortilla chips

And some combination of:
black beans
refried beans
diced white onion
sliced black olives
sliced jalapeños
cilantro

Preheat your oven to 350, cause we're going to bake this baby for maximum cohesion and warm deliciousness.

Start with a casserole pan or baking sheet of whatever size you need to hold your pile of nachos. It's important to construct the nacho pile using a layering technique to ensure an even distribution of ingredients, so that each bite will be as enjoyable as the last. Layer in everything except the guacamole, which doesn't want to be baked. End with your cheese sauce on top.

Bake uncovered for fifteen-twenty minutes to heat everything thoroughly and firm up the cheese layer on top. Slop on some guacamole and dig in!

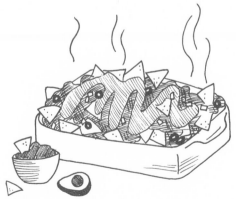

Arroz con Leche

This was a special request from my partner José, who has assured me it is up to par after generously agreeing to taste-test it again and again. One torturous taste-test after another found it to be delicately sweet and flavorful, with just a hint of cinnamon and the barely detectable addition of creamy coconut milk.

Serves: 4

1 can (14oz.) light coconut milk
2 1/4 cup soymilk
1/2 cup short grain white rice (I've had good success with sushi rice)
1/2 tsp salt
1 cinnamon stick
1/2 cup sugar
2 Tbsp vegan margarine
1 tsp vanilla
ground cinnamon for garnish

Combine coconut milk, soymilk, rice, salt, and cinnamon stick in a covered pot and bring to a boil. Once boiling, immediately reduce to very low heat and allow the mixture to simmer for fourty five minutes. Stir often and be sure to scrape the bottom so it doesn't burn.

After fourty five minutes, mix in the sugar, margarine, and vanilla and take the lid off of your pot for the remainder of the cooking time. Keep stirring and allow to simmer for fifteen more minutes.

Dish it up and sprinkle with some ground cinnamon and you're done!

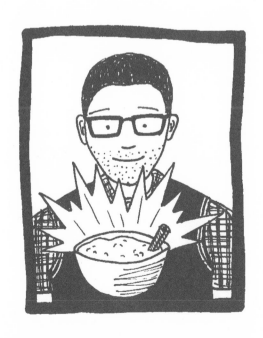

Barley Salad with Cranberries and Arugula

This recipe is based on a prepared dish I once found at the salad bar of my local grocery store. I was impressed at the use of barley in a salad and bought a small serving of it. Lo and behold, it was damn good! It had a good mixture of sweetness and savory elements, plus the brightness of citrus. I had to replicate it. So here you go, barley salad from the market to me, and from me to you.

Serves: 4-6

1 cup pearled barley
3 cup water
1/2 cup red onion, very thinly sliced
1/3 cup chopped pecans (or walnuts, if you can't get your hands on pecans)
1/3 cup dried cranberries
1 cup arugula, or more if you're a big fan!

For the dressing:
1/3 cup orange juice
1 Tbsp olive oil
1 Tbsp apple cider vinegar
1/4 tsp salt
1/4 tsp pepper

Cook your barley. Bring the water to a boil, then add in barley and reduce the heat. Barley cooks like rice, just for a slightly longer time. Cover and cook for about 35 minutes until it is tender, stirring a couple times throughout.

Remove from heat and let the barley sit uncovered, or transfer to the fridge while you prepare the rest of your ingredients. For this recipe, I like my barley to be warm, not hot, when I assemble the salad, but you can try it however you like, from stovetop-hot to refrigerator-cold and see what you prefer!

Chop your onion and pecans, and then work on putting together your dressing. Whisk all the dressing ingredients together in a glass or small bowl.

Once the barley is at your desired level of warmness or coolness, toss in the other salad ingredients and then the dressing. Add more salt and pepper to taste if you like.

Perfect Popcorn

In some ways a non-recipe, I had to include it in here to spread the secret to perfect popcorn! I can't help myself, and I hope snacking will be better off for it. This one goes out to my cat, GG, who thoroughly enjoys licking the nutritional yeast out of the bowl once all the perfect popcorn is gone.

Serves: 2-4

1/2 cup or so unpopped popcorn kernels
a couple Tbsp melted vegan margarine
salt
garlic powder
tons of nutritional yeast

Pop your popcorn however you prefer (air popper, stovetop, microwave). Melt your margarine and drizzle over the popped popcorn in batches to get an even coating. Sprinkle with salt and dust generously with garlic powder. Coat the whole thing with a handful of nutritional yeast. The yeast, salt and garlic powder will stick to the margarine, so you should be able to get a nice coating.

Serves 2 to 4, but I bet you could eat it all yourself if you really tried. I believe in you!

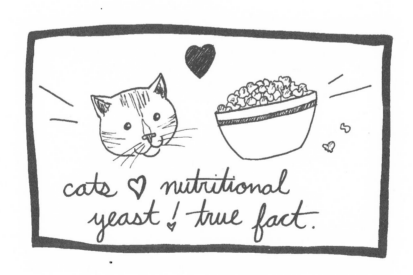

Brown Sugar Caramel Corn

Perfect popcorn's sweet cousin, this caramel corn is a snack of a different stripe. Brown sugar gives the popcorn a deep, rich sweetness without being *overly* sweet, and has enough salt to compliment the sugar nicely. Also, it's easy and fun to make. You'll never need to buy kettle corn from the fair or farmer's market again!

Makes: up to 6 cups

1/4 cup canola oil
1/2 cup unpopped popcorn kernels
1/3 cup brown sugar
pinch of salt

In a large, heavy, lidded pan, heat up your canola oil on high for two to three minutes. Once it's nice and hot, add the popcorn kernels and salt. Turn the heat down to medium, put the lid on, and start shaking. Give the pot a good shake every thirty seconds or so. Heat the popcorn for about three minutes (it will have started popping by this point) before adding in your brown sugar. Put the sugar in, put the lid back on, and shake it some more. Keep shaking (good exercise, right? You're gonna earn this shit) and continue to pop over medium heat for another five minutes or so. By now you should only be getting pops every couple seconds. Remove from heat and continue to shake for a minute until all the popping has stopped. Now transfer to a large bowl to cool off, and stir with a fork to break up big clumps. You did it!

Savory Sautéed Brussels with Shallots

One of my favorite preparations of brussels sprouts serves well over a bed of angel hair pasta with just a little margarine or olive oil and garlic. Tons of veggies; tons of flavor; not a ton of work. Another great introduction for folks who think they hate brussels sprouts. Can you tell I'm on a mission to save the reputation of one of my favorite veggies here?

Serves: 2-4

1 lb (~3-4 cup whole) brussels sprouts
1 shallot, minced
2 Tbsp pine nuts (optional-ish—if you really can't get 'em, it's ok)
2 Tbsp olive oil
1 Tbsp Braggs liquid aminos, plus some more to taste, if you like
salt and pepper to taste

Chop the Brussels sprouts, first in half, and then into shreds long-ways, like the diagram. Mince your shallot, then toss together brussels shreds, shallot, olive oil and Braggs in a large pan. Cook over medium heat, stirring constantly, for twelve to fourteen minutes. Toss in your pine nuts for the last couple minutes of cooking, and sprinkle in salt and pepper to taste.

Serve over a bed of angel hair pasta (about one fourth to one third of a sixteen oz. package will compliment this recipe).

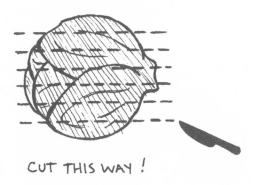

CUT THIS WAY !

Apple Cinnamon Breakfast Quinoa

Quinoa being pretty close to the perfect food and all, it makes sense to try and incorporate it into your diet wherever you can. And lucky for us, it makes sense as a lovely hot breakfast cereal, aided by tasty cooked apples and a bit of cinnamon and sugar. Think of it as oatmeal's tough-but-sweet powerhouse of a cousin.

Serves: up to 4

1 cup quinoa
2 cup soymilk
1 small apple, diced small (about 3/4 cup diced)
1/2 tsp cinnamon
1 Tbsp brown sugar

Optional toppings:
dried fruit
nuts
extra soymilk

Bring soymilk, quinoa, sugar and cinnamon to boil on the stove, then reduce heat to low. Cook for ten minutes before adding in your apple chunks. Stir every few minutes to keep the quinoa from sticking to the bottom of the pan. You can go ahead and peel and cut up the apples during this time for extra efficiency.

Toss in the apples and continue to simmer for another fifteen minutes, continuing to stir every so often. Your apples and quinoa should be tender and the soymilk completely absorbed when you're done.

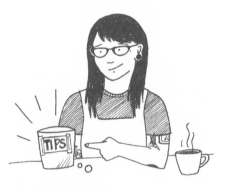

*Ridiculously useful tip:
Serve your breakfast quinoa as is, top it with dried fruit and nuts for a crunchy, hearty treat, or forego the toppings and pour a little soymilk over it for a comforting, creamy meal.

Stuffed Acorn Squash

A super-impressive side dish, or a satisfying main dish, acorn squash are hearty, delicious, and perfect for fall! The nuts and cranberries in the filling give a variety of textures with bursts of crunch and sweetness. The acorn squash itself is delicate and delicious. Enjoy these topped with You'd-Never-Know-It-Was-Vegan Gravy and a side of Brussels sprouts!

Serves: 4

2 medium acorn squash
1 Tbsp olive oil

For the filling:
1/2 cup brown rice
1/4 cup wild rice
1 3/4 cup vegetable broth (or hot water + 1 bouillon cube)
1/2 cup chopped walnuts
1/4 cup dried cranberries, coarsely chopped

One recipe You'd-Never-Know-It-Was-Vegan Gravy (pg. 24)

Preheat your oven to 400. Cut your acorn squash in half long-ways, from stem to base. Scoop out the seeds with a spoon and toss 'em. Coat the cut surface of the squash with a little olive oil and place face-down in a casserole pan. Roast for about twenty five minutes until they are tender and piercable with a fork.

In the meantime, prepare your filling! Combine the two types of rice and the veg broth in a rice cooker and cook until done, about twenty minutes. If you don't have a rice cooker, simmer on low, stirring occasionally until all liquid is absorbed and the rice is tender.

While your squash is in the oven, take the opportunity to toast your walnut pieces! Roasting nuts brings out a nice flavor and aroma, and only takes a few minutes. Just toss them in the oven on a baking sheet or tinfoil for five to seven minutes.

When your rice is cooked and the nuts are toasted, combine all the filling ingredients.

Your squash should be just about done. Take them out of the oven and flip over. Fill each with a generous scoop of the filling and put them back in their pan. Spoon some gravy over the tops and return to the oven for ten more minutes or so. Enjoy!

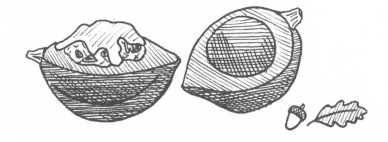

About the Author

Ashley Rowe grew up in Los Angeles and came to veganism more than a dozen years ago through the radical politics of the punk scene. She started cooking while in high school and put out the first issue of the *Barefoot and in the Kitchen* zine a few years later, while living and attending college in Santa Cruz.

Ashley currently lives, loves, cooks and works in Oakland, CA, where she is co-owner of the all-vegan Fat Bottom Bakery.

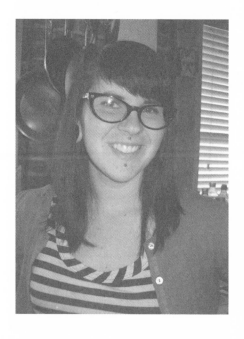

Acknowledgments

Many thanks to the following for all your support, love, inspiration, and contributions:

José Palafox, Kathleen Rubio, Jessie Fun Punx, Laura Beck and the rest of the Vegansaurus crew, Tucker Zappas, Jang Lee, Under and Willy Bananas, and all my other friends with inspiring bands, businesses and projects.

Speaking of inspiring individuals, I want to give thanks especially to all my wonderful friends who contributed guest recipes: Carolynn Webb, Camelia Rivera and Mariana Palafox, Tamar Shirinian, Seth Kramer, Debbie Nguyen, Gina Giarrusso, and Lorna Vetters.

My family, for their acceptance and encouragement of all my choices and ventures: Tom and Jill Rowe, Justin Rowe, Barbara McCurry, and Nancy Kersnowski.

Everyone at Microcosm Publishing—past and present—for supporting this project when it started as a zine and now that it's grown into a full-fledged book.

AK Press, for being such an incredible source of information and inspiration—and for being full of rad folks).
www.akpress.org

Anyone who's ever bought, traded, or otherwise picked up the *Barefoot* zine, and especially those of you who've gotten in touch with me to talk about it. I'm so happy to have had the opportunity to trade skills and ideas with so many great people over the years, and to hear all the stories of new vegans and satisfied omnivores who've gotten to enjoy a new recipe or two.

BE OUR "BEST FRIEND FOREVER"

Do you love what Microcosm publishes?
Do you want us to publish more great stuff?
Would you like to receive each new title as
it's published?

If you answer "yes!" then you should subscribe
to our BFF program. BFF subscribers help
pay for printing new books, zines, and more.
They also ensure that we can continue to
print great material each month! Every time
we publish something new we'll send it to
your door!

Subscriptions are based on a sliding scale
of $10-30 per month. Please give what you
can afford so that we can be sure to send
out more stuff each month. Include your
t-shirt size and month/date of birthday for
a possible surprise!

Minimum subscription period is 6 months. Subscription begins the month after
it is purchased. To receive more than 6 months, add multiple orders to your
quantity.

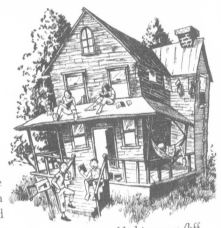

microcosmpublishing.com/bff

Microcosm Publishing
636 SE 11th Ave. Portland, OR 97214
www.microcosmpublishing.com